Air Fryer Cookbook
for Beginners

Almost 300 Delicious Recipes, Using Just Your Air Fryer. 21 Days Meal Plan Included.

Table of Contents

Introduction to the air fryer

What are advantages of Cosori Air Fryer

In the long run, The Cosori Air Fryer will significantly cut down your Oil Intake, in fact, researches have shown that it has the capacity to cut it down by almost 80%! This is possibly the healthiest advantage that you will experience while using an Air Fryer. However, if you want to go even further:

- Prepare awesome and extremely delicious meals without any hassle

- Unlike most other bulky cooking appliances, cleaning the Cosori is extremely easy (as seen the next segment

- Since the Air Fryer helps to cut down oil, cooking with the Fryer will significantly contribute in weight loss and allow you to stay healthy

- If you are in a rush, the Air Fryer will greatly be advantageous to you as well since it allows you to cook extremely fast!

Learning to Keep Your Device Clean

Just like any other cooking appliance, the Cosori also has the potential accumulate dirt and debris as you keep using it for prolonged period of time. If you don't take care of it properly, the appliance's life might get reduced. Therefore, it is highly advised that you keep your appliance as much clean as possible to get the best experience out of it.

The following simple steps should help you keep your Fryer clean with ease.

- It is very normal for meals to leave a sticky residue inside the cooking basket of the fryer. An easy way to deal with this is to use specialized detergents or soap that are designed to dissolve oil.

- For maximum effect, try to soak the detergent mixed water for a few minutes before thoroughly rinsing it under hot water.

- Always keep in mind that metal utensils and cleaning brushes may leave scratches on the body of the Fryer. So, refrain yourself from using those.

- Make sure to complete cool down your Air Fryer and wait for 30 minutes prior to washing it

And on the topic of cleaning, you should remember the following steps while cleaning up your appliance:

- Remove the power cable from the wall and make sure that the device is completely cooled.

- Wipe out the external part of the Fryer using a moist cloth dipped in mild detergent.

- Clean the outer basket and the fryer basket and using hot water (mixed with mild detergentand a soft sponge.

- Clean the inner part of the appliance using hot water (with mild detergentand a soft sponge.

- If you find that some residue is stuck in the heating element, then you may use a cleaning brush to clear them out.

Understanding the Science behind Air Fryer

Since you will be spending a lot of time with this appliance, perhaps it would be wise if you knew how the Air Fryer process actually works right?

Well, it's pretty simple if you think about it.

The keyword here is "Air"

Most other conventional cooking appliances tend to cook their meal by using some sort of heater that passes heat through the meal through a process known as conduction. This basically transfer heat to the meal on touch.

An Air Fryer on the other hand, does its cooking through a process called "Convection" where air is heated up and circulated throughout the food.

During your journey into the various super markets looking for an Air Fryer, you have most definitely seen the word "Rapid Air Technology" countless times. That actually refers to a very delicately designed process which the Air Fryer uses to cook its food.

The Air Is sucked up the intake chamber and the appliance gets heated up.

Chapter 1. Breakfast recipes

1. Peppery Sausage & Parsley Patties

Preparation Time: 20 minutes
Servings: 4

Ingredients

1 lb ground Italian sausage

¼ cup breadcrumbs

1 tsp dried parsley

1 tsp red pepper flakes

½ tsp salt

¼ tsp black pepper

¼ tsp garlic powder

1 egg, beaten

Directions

Preheat the air fryer to 350 degrees F. Combine all of the ingredients in a large bowl. Line a baking sheet with parchment paper. Make patties out of the sausage mixture and arrange them on the baking sheet. Cook for 15 minutes, flipping once halfway through cooking.

2. Air Fried Mac and Cheese

Preparation Time: 15 minutes
Servings: 2

Ingredients

1 cup cooked macaroni

1 cup grated cheddar cheese

½ cup warm milk

1 tbsp Parmesan cheese

Salt and black pepper to taste

Directions

Preheat the air fryer to 350 degrees F. Add the macaroni to an ovenproof baking dish. Stir in the cheddar and milk. Season with salt and pepper, to taste. Place the dish in the air fryer and cook for 10 minutes. Sprinkle with Parmesan cheese, to serve.

3. Prosciutto & Mozzarella Crostini

Preparation Time: 7 minutes
Servings: 1

Ingredients

½ cup finely chopped tomatoes

3 oz chopped mozzarella

3 prosciutto slices, chopped

1 tbsp olive oil

1 tsp dried basil

6 small slices of French bread

Directions

Preheat the air fryer to 350 degrees F. Place the bread slices and toast for 3 minutes. Top the bread with tomatoes, prosciutto and mozzarella. Sprinkle the basil over the mozzarella. Drizzle with olive oil. Return to the air fryer and cook for 1 more minute, enough to become melty and warm.

4. Vanilla Lemon Cheesecake

Preparation Time: 80 minutes + chilling time
Servings: 8

Ingredients

8 oz graham crackers, crushed

4 oz butter, melted

16 oz plain cream cheese

3 eggs

3 tbsp sugar

1 tbsp vanilla extract

Zest of 2 lemons

Directions

Line a cake tin, that fits in your Air fryer, with baking paper. Mix together the crackers and butter, and press at the bottom of the tin. In a bowl, add cream cheese, eggs, sugar, vanilla and lemon zest and beat with a hand mixer until well combined and smooth. Pour the mixture into the tin, on top of the cracker's base. Cook for 40-45 minutes at 350 F, checking it to ensure it's set but still a bit wobbly. Let cool, then refrigerate overnight.

5. Cinnamon Baked Apples with Raisins & Walnuts

Preparation Time: 35 minutes
Servings: 2

Ingredients

2 granny smith apples, cored, bottom intact

2 tbsp butter, cold

3 tbsp sugar

3 tbsp crushed walnuts

2 tbsp raisins

1 tsp cinnamon

Directions

In a bowl, add butter, sugar, walnuts, raisins and cinnamon; mix with fingers until you obtain a crumble. Arrange the apples in the Air fryer. Stuff the apples with the filling mixture. Cook for 30 minutes at 400 F.

6. Vanilla Chocolate Brownies with Walnuts

Preparation Time: 35 minutes
Servings: 10

Ingredients

6 oz dark chocolate

6 oz butter

¾ cup white sugar

3 eggs

2 tsp vanilla extract

¾ cup flour

¼ cup cocoa powder

1 cup chopped walnuts

1 cup white chocolate chips

Directions

Line a pan inside your Air fryer with baking paper. In a saucepan, melt chocolate and butter over low heat. Do not stop stirring until you obtain a smooth mixture. Let cool slightly, whisk in eggs and vanilla. Sift flour and cocoa and stir to mix well. Sprinkle the walnuts over and add the white chocolate into the batter. Pour the batter into the pan and cook for 20 minutes at 340 F. Serve with raspberry syrup and ice cream.

7. Raspberry Chocolate Cake

Preparation Time: 40 minutes
Servings: 8

Ingredients

1 ½ cups flour

⅓ cup cocoa powder

2 tsp baking powder

¾ cup white sugar

¼ cup brown sugar

⅔ cup butter

2 tsp vanilla extract

1 cup milk

1 tsp baking soda

2 eggs

1 cup freeze-dried raspberries

1 cup chocolate chips

Directions

Line a cake tin with baking powder. In a bowl, sift flour, cocoa and baking powder. Place the sugars, butter, vanilla, milk and baking soda into a microwave-safe bowl and heat for 60 seconds until the butter melts and the ingredients incorporate; let cool slightly. Whisk the eggs into the mixture.

Pour the wet ingredients into the dry ones, and fold to combine. Add in the raspberries and chocolate chips into the batter. Pour the batter into the tin and cook for 30 minutes at 350 F.

8. Amazing Marshmallows Pie

Preparation Time: 10 minutes
Servings: 4

Ingredients

4 graham cracker sheets, snapped in half

8 large marshmallows

8 squares each of dark, milk and white chocolate

Directions

Arrange the cracker halves on a board. Put 2 marshmallows onto half of the graham cracker halves. Place 2 squares of chocolate onto the cracker with the marshmallows. Put the remaining crackers on top to create 4 sandwiches. Wrap each one in the baking paper so it resembles a parcel. Cook in the fryer for 5 minutes at 340 F.

9. Caramel Apple & Cinnamon Cake

Preparation Time: 40 minutes
Servings: 4

Ingredients

1 vanilla box cake

2 apples, peeled, sliced

3 oz butter, melted

½ cup brown sugar

1 tsp cinnamon

½ cup flour

1 cup caramel sauce

Directions

Line a cake tin with baking paper. In a bowl, mix butter, sugar, cinnamon and flour until you obtain a crumbly texture. Prepare the cake mix according to the instructions (no baking). Pour the batter into the tin and arrange the apple slices on top. Spoon the caramel over the apples and add the crumble over the sauce. Cook in the Air fryer for 35 minutes at 360 F; make sure to check it halfway through, so it's not overcooked.

10. Marshmallows Choco S´mores

Preparation Time: 10 minutes
Servings: 4

Ingredients

4 graham cracker sheets, snapped in half

8 large marshmallows

8 squares each of dark, milk and white chocolate

Directions

Arrange the cracker halves on a board. Put 2 marshmallows onto half of the graham cracker halves. Place 2 squares of chocolate onto the cracker with the marshmallows. Put the remaining crackers on top to create 4 sandwiches. Wrap each one in baking paper so it resembles a parcel. Place in your Air fryer and cook for 5 minutes at 340 F.

11. Delicious Figs with Honey & Mascarpone

Preparation Time: 10 minutes
Servings: 4

INGREDIENTS

8 figs

6 oz mascarpone cheese

1 tsp rose water

1 oz butter

3 tbsp honey

2 tbsp toasted almond slices

DIRECTIONS

Preheat the Air fryer to 350 F, open the figs by cutting a cross on top and gently squeezing them. Divide the honey between the figs. Place them on a lined baking sheet and cook for 5 minutes. Combine the mascarpone with the rose water. Place a dollop of the mascarpone onto each fig, top with toasted almonds and serve.

12. Dark Chocolate & Peanut Butter Fondant

Preparation Time: 25 minutes
Servings: 4

Ingredients

¾ cup dark chocolate

½ cup peanut butter, crunchy

2 tbsp butter, diced

¼ cup + ¼ cup sugar

4 eggs, room temperature

⅛ cup flour, sieved

1 tsp salt

¼ cup water

Directions

Make a salted praline to top the chocolate fondant. Add ¼ cup of sugar, 1 tsp of salt and water into a saucepan. Stir and bring it to a boil over low heat on a stove top. Simmer until the desired color is achieved and reduced.

Pour it into a baking tray and leave to cool and harden. Preheat the Air Fryer to 300 F. Place a pot of water over medium heat and place a heatproof bowl over it. Add the chocolate, butter, and peanut butter to the bowl.

Stir continuously until fully melted, combined, and smooth. Remove the bowl from the heat and allow to cool slightly. Add the eggs to the chocolate and whisk. Add the flour and remaining sugar; mix well.

Grease 4 small loaf pans with cooking spray and divide the chocolate mixture between them. Place 2 pans at a time in the basket and cook for 7 minutes. Remove them and serve the fondants with a piece of salted praline.

13. Dreamy White Chocolate Dessert

Preparation Time: 40 minutes
Servings: 2

Ingredients

3 oz white chocolate

4 large egg whites

2 large egg yolks, at room temperature

¼ cup sugar + more for garnishing

1 tbsp melted butter

1 tbsp unmelted butter

¼ tsp vanilla extract

1 ½ tbsp flour

Directions

Coat two 6-oz ramekins with melted butter. Add the sugar and swirl it in the ramekins to coat the butter. Pour out the remaining sugar and keep it. Melt the unmelted butter with the chocolate in a microwave; set aside.

In another bowl, beat the egg yolks vigorously. Add the vanilla and kept sugar; beat to incorporate fully. Add the chocolate mixture and mix well. Add the flour and mix it with no lumps.

Preheat the Air Fryer to 330 F, and whisk the egg whites in another bowl till it holds stiff peaks. Add ⅓ of the egg whites into the chocolate mixture; fold in gently and evenly. Share the mixture into the ramekins with ½ inch space left at the top. Place the ramekins in the fryer basket, close the Air Fryer and cook for 14 minutes.

Dust with the remaining sugar and serve.

14. Homemade Orange Curd

Preparation Time: 30 minutes
Servings: 2

Ingredients

3 tbsp butter

3 tbsp sugar

1 egg

1 egg yolk

¾ orange, juiced

Directions

Add sugar and butter in a medium ramekin and beat evenly. Add egg and yolk slowly while still whisking. the fresh yellow color will be attained. Add the orange juice and mix. Place the bowl in the fryer basket and cook at 250 F for 6 minutes. Increase the temperature again to 320 F and cook for 15 minutes.

Remove the bowl onto a flat surface; use a spoon to check for any lumps and remove. Cover the ramekin with a plastic wrap and refrigerate overnight or serve immediately.

15. Tasty Choco-Banana Sandwich

Preparation Time: 30 minutes
Servings: 2

Ingredients

4 slices of brioche

1 tbsp butter, melted

6 oz milk chocolate, broken into chunks

1 banana, sliced

Directions

Brush the brioche slices with butter. Spread chocolate and banana on 2 brioche slices. Top with the remaining 2 slices to create 2 sandwiches. Arrange the sandwiches into your air fryer and cook for 14 minutes at 400 F, turning once halfway through. Slice in half and serve with vanilla ice cream.

16. Vanilla Crème Caramel

Preparation Time: 60 minutes
Servings: 3

Ingredients

1 cup whipped cream

1 cup milk

2 vanilla pods

10 egg yolks

4 tbsp sugar + extra for topping

Directions

In a pan, add the milk and cream. Cut the vanilla pods open and scrape the seeds into the pan with the vanilla pods also. Place the pan over medium heat on a stove top until almost boiled while stirring regularly. Turn off the heat. Add the egg yolks to a bowl and beat it. Add the sugar and mix well but not too frothy.

Remove the vanilla pods from the milk mixture; pour the mixture onto the eggs mixture while stirring constantly. Let it sit for 25 minutes. Fill 2 to 3 ramekins with the mixture. Place the ramekins in the fryer basket and cook them at 190 F for 50 minutes. Once ready, remove the ramekins and let sit to cool. Sprinkle the remaining sugar over and use a torch to melt the sugar, so it browns at the top.

17. Orange & Chocolate Fudge with Honey Icing

Preparation Time: 55 minutes
Servings: 8

Ingredients

1 cup sugar

7 oz flour

1 tbsp honey

¼ cup milk

1 tsp vanilla extract

1 oz cocoa powder

2 eggs

4 oz butter

1 orange, juice and zest

Icing:

1 oz butter, melted

4 oz powdered sugar

1 tbsp brown sugar

1 tbsp milk

2 tsp honey

Directions

Preheat the Air fryer to 350 F, and in a bowl, mix the dry ingredients for the fudge. Mix the wet ingredients separately; combine the two mixtures gently. Transfer the batter to a prepared cake pan. Cook for 35 minutes. Meanwhile whisk together all icing ingredients. When the cake cools, coat with the icing. Let set before slicing.

18. Coconut Oat Cookies Filled with White Chocolate

Preparation Time: 30 minutes
Servings: 4

Ingredients

5 ½ oz flour

1 tsp vanilla extract

3 oz sugar

½ cup oats

1 small egg, beaten

¼ cup coconut flakes

Filling:

1 oz white chocolate, melted

2 oz butter

4 oz powdered sugar

1 tsp vanilla extract

Directions

Beat all the cookie ingredients, with an electric mixer, except the flour.
When smooth, fold in the flour. Drop spoonfuls of the batter onto a prepared
cookie sheet. Cook in the Air fryer at 350 F for 18 minutes; then let cool.

Meanwhile, prepare the filling by beating all ingredients together; spread the
filling on half of the cookies. Top with the other halves to make cookie
sandwiches.

19. Honeyed White Chocolate Cake

Preparation Time: 30 minutes
Servings: 8

Ingredients

6 oz self-rising flour

3 oz brown sugar

2 oz white chocolate chips

1 tbsp honey

1 ½ tbsp milk

4 oz butter

Directions

Preheat the Air fryer to 350 F, and beat the butter and sugar until fluffy.
Beat in the honey, milk, and flour. Gently fold in the chocolate chips. Drop
spoonfuls of the mixture onto a prepared cookie sheet. Cook for 18 minutes.

20. Blueberry & Yogurt Cups

Preparation Time: 30 minutes
Servings: 10

Ingredients

1 ½ cup flour

½ tsp salt

½ cup sugar

¼ cup vegetable oil

2 tsp vanilla extract

1 cup blueberries

1 egg

2 tsp baking powder

Yogurt, as needed

Directions

Preheat the Air fryer to 350 F, and combine flour, salt and baking powder, in a bowl. In another bowl, add the oil, vanilla extract, and egg. Fill the rest of the bowl with yogurt, and whisk the mixture until fully incorporated.

Combine the wet and dry ingredients; gently fold in the blueberries. Divide the mixture between 10 muffin cups. You may need to work in batches. Cook for 10 minutes.

21. Creamy Yogurt & Lime Muffins

Preparation Time: 30 minutes
Servings: 6

Ingredients

2 eggs plus 1 yolk

Juice and zest of 2 limes

1 cup yogurt

¼ cup superfine sugar

8 oz cream cheese

1 tsp vanilla extract

Directions

Preheat the Air fryer to 330 F, and with a spatula, gently combine the yogurt and cheese. In another bowl, beat together the rest of the ingredients. Gently fold the lime with the cheese mixture. Divide the batter between 6 lined muffin tins. Cook in the Air fryer for 10 minutes.

22. Easy Cinnamon Snickerdoodle Cookies

Preparation Time: 30 minutes
Servings: 6

Ingredients

1 box instant vanilla Jell-O

1 can of Pillsbury Grands Flaky Layers Biscuits

1 ½ cups cinnamon sugar

melted butter, for brushing

Directions

Preheat the Air fryer to 350 F, and unroll the flaky biscuits; cut them into fourths. Roll each ¼ into a ball. Arrange the balls on a lined baking sheet, and cook in the air fryer for 7 minutes, or until golden.

Meanwhile, prepare the Jell-O following the package's instructions. Using an injector, inject some of the vanilla pudding into each ball. Brush the balls with melted butter and then coat them with cinnamon sugar.

23. Foolproof Cherry Pie

Preparation Time: 30 minutes
Servings: 8

Ingredients

2 store-bought pie crusts

21 oz cherry pie filling

1 egg yolk

1 tbsp milk

Directions

Preheat the Air fryer to 310 F, and place one pie crust in a pie pan; poke holes into the crust. Cook for 5 minutes.

Spread the pie filling over. Cut the other pie crust into strips and arrange the pie-style over the baked crust.

Whisk milk and egg yolk, and brush the mixture over the pie. Return the pie to the fryer and cook for 15 minutes.

24. Vanilla & Chocolate Chip Cookies

Preparation Time: 15 minutes
Servings: 5

Ingredients

¾ cup flour

¼ tsp baking soda

¾ tsp salt

⅓ cup brown sugar

¼ cup unsalted butter, softened

2 tbsp white sugar

1 egg yolk

½ tbsp vanilla extract

½ cup chocolate chips

Directions

Preheat air fryer to 350 F. Line the basket or rack with foil. Whisk flour, baking soda, and salt together in a small bowl. Combine brown sugar, butter, and white sugar in a separate bowl.

Add egg yolk and vanilla extract and whisk until well-combined. Stir flour mixture into butter mixture until dough is just combined; gently fold in chocolate chips. Scoop dough by the spoonfuls and roll into balls; place onto the foil-lined air fryer basket, 2 inches apart.

Cook dough in the air fryer until cookies start getting crispy, 5 to 6 minutes. Transfer foil and cookies to wire racks or a plate, and let cool completely. Repeat with remaining dough.

25. Banana Fritters

Preparation Time: 6 minutes
Servings: 6

INGREDIENTS

6 bananas

4 large eggs, beaten

1 cup breadcrumbs

1 cup bread flour

1 cup oil

DIRECTIONS

Peel the bananas and cut them into pieces of less than 1-inch each. In a bowl, mix the beaten eggs with the bread flour and the oil. Dredge the banana first into the flour, then dip in the beaten eggs, and finally in the crumbs. Line the banana pieces in the Air Fryer and cook them for 10 minutes at 350° F, shaking once halfway through. Serve with vanilla ice cream.

26. Pineapple Chocolate Cake

Preparation Time: 50 minutes
Servings: 4

Ingredients

2 oz dark chocolate, grated

8 oz self-rising flour

4 oz butter

7 oz pineapple chunks

½ cup pineapple juice

1 egg

2 tbsp milk

½ cup sugar

Directions

Preheat the Air fryer to 390 F, place the butter and flour into a bowl, and rub the mixture with your fingers until crumbed. Stir in pineapple, sugar, chocolate, and juice. Beat eggs and milk separately, and then add to the batter.

Transfer the batter to a previously prepared (greased or linedcake pan, and cook for 40 minutes. Let cool for at least 10 minutes before serving.

27. Grandma's Buttermilk Biscuits

Preparation Time: 25 minutes
Servings: 4

Ingredients

1 ¼ cups flour, plus some for dusting

½ tsp baking soda

½ cup cake flour

¾ tsp salt

½ tsp baking powder

4 tbsp butter, chopped

1 tsp sugar

¾ cup buttermilk

Directions

Preheat the Air fryer to 400 F and combine all dry ingredients, in a bowl. Place the chopped butter in the bowl, and rub it into the flour mixture, until crumbed. Stir in the buttermilk.

Flour a flat and dry surface and roll out until half-inch thick. Cut out 10 rounds with a small cookie cutter. Arrange the biscuits on a lined baking sheet. Cook for 8 minutes.

28. Homemade Doughnuts

Preparation Time: 25 minutes
Servings: 4

Ingredients

8 oz self-rising flour

1 tsp baking powder

½ cup milk

2 ½ tbsp butter

1 egg

2 oz brown sugar

Directions

Preheat the Air fryer to 350 F, and beat the butter with the sugar, until smooth. Beat in eggs, and milk. In a bowl, combine the flour with the baking powder. Gently fold the flour into the butter mixture.

Form donut shapes and cut off the center with cookie cutters. Arrange on a lined baking sheet and cook in the fryer for 15 minutes. Serve with whipped cream or icing.

29. Glazed Lemon Cupcakes

Preparation Time: 30 minutes
Servings: 6

Ingredients

1 cup flour

½ cup sugar

1 small egg

1 tsp lemon zest

¾ tsp baking powder

¼ tsp baking soda

½ tsp salt

2 tbsp vegetable oil

½ cup milk

½ tsp vanilla extract

Glaze:

½ cup powdered sugar

2 tsp lemon juice

Directions

Preheat the Air fryer to 350 F, and combine all dry muffin ingredients, in a bowl. In another bowl, whisk together the wet ingredients. Gently combine the two mixtures. Divide the batter between 6 greased muffin tins.

Place the muffin tins in the Air fryer and cook for 12 to 14 minutes. Meanwhile, whisk the powdered sugar with the lemon juice. Spread the glaze over the muffins.

30. Air Fryer Whole Chicken

Preparation Time: 5 minutes

Cooking Time: 40 minutes

Servings: 8

Nutrition:

Calories: 336

Protein: 25.42 g

Fat: 23.86 g

Carbs: 3.72 g

Ingredients:

1 whole chicken

2 sliced tomatoes

1 sliced onion

1 cup yogurt

1 tsp. salt

2 tbsps. olive oil

½ tsp. chili powder

½ tsp. cinnamon powder

1 tsp. garlic powder

2 tbsps. lime juice

1 tsp. vinegar

Directions

In a bowl add yogurt, salt, chili powder, garlic powder, cinnamon powder, lime juice, vinegar, and olive oil, mix.

Drizzle yogurt sauce over chicken and rub all over.

Preheat Air Fryer at the temperature of 370°F.

Place onion and tomatoes inside the chicken.

Transfer chicken into fryer basket and cook for about 20 minutes.

After that turn chicken and cook again for 20 minutes.

Serve.

31. Cauliflower BBQ with Honey and Mayo Sauce

Preparation Time: 5 minutes

Cooking Time: 12 minutes

Servings: 4

Nutrition:

Calories: 276

Protein: 5.49 g

Fat: 11.52 g

Carbs: 39.45 g

Ingredients:

1 cup all-purpose flour

3 cs. cauliflower, florets

1 tsp. salt

¼ tsp. smoked paprika

½ tsp. cinnamon powder

½ tsp. cumin powder

1 cup mayonnaise

1 tsp. chili powder

1 tsp. onion powder

1 tsp. garlic powder

Directions:

Preheat your Air Fryer to a temperature of 400°F.

In a bowl add flour, salt, chili powder, cumin powder, cinnamon powder, and onion powder, mix well.

Add 5 tbsps. of water and make a thick batter.

Add in cauliflower florets and coat well.

Spray fryer basket with some oil.

Now place cauliflower florets into fryer basket and cook for 6 minutes.

After that turn side and cook for another 6 minutes.

In a bowl add mayonnaise, smoked paprika, and garlic powder, mix well.

Serve BBQ cauliflower with your favorite vegetables.

32. Air Fryer Chicken Wings with Olives

Preparation Time: 10 minutes

Cooking Time: 30 minutes

Servings: 4

Nutrition:

Calories: 344

Fat: 14.5g

Carbs: 1.4g

Protein: 49.4g

Ingredients:

1½ lbs. chicken wings

½ cup olives

1 tsp. oregano

1½ tsps. lemon juice

Salt

Garlic powder

Directions:

Mix to combine salt, lemon juice, garlic powder, and oregano in a bowl.

Add the meat and toss until coated.

Arrange half of the seasoned meat in the cooking basket.

Cook for 10 minutes at 3560F.

Shake the basket twice during the process.

Add the olives and cook for 5 more minutes.

Perform the same cooking process with the remaining chicken wings.

Serve while hot.

33. Chicken Nuggets

Preparation Time: 20 minutes

Cooking Time: 25 minutes

Servings: 4

Nutrition:

Calories: 356

Fat: 9.3g

Carbohydrates: 27.2g

Protein: 38.2g

Ingredients:

1 lb. chopped chicken breasts

1 cup flour

1 cup buttermilk

1 tsp. salt

½ tsp. garlic powder

½ tsp. paprika

Directions:

Set the meat in a big bowl and cover with buttermilk to marinate for one hour.

Combine paprika, mix flour, salt, and garlic powder in a bowl.

Add the meat and toss until coated. Arrange 8 chicken nuggets in the cooking basket at a time. Lightly spray them with oil.

Cook for 10 minutes at 400 degrees.

Set on a platter then cook the remaining nuggets.

Serve and enjoy.

34. Spicy Chicken Fajitas

Preparation Time: 13 minutes

Cooking Time: 21 minutes

Servings: 4

Nutrition:

Calories: 426

Fat: 20.1g

Carbs: 21.5g

Protein: 40g

Ingredients:

1 lb. chicken breasts

1 chopped onion

1 sliced green pepper

1 sliced red pepper

½ tsp. chili powder

½ tsp. ground coriander

1 tsp. garlic powder

½ tsp. sea salt

¼ tsp. ground cumin

¼ tsp. ground black pepper

1 tbsp. fresh lime juice

For garnishing:

½ cup shredded cheddar cheese

½ cup medium salsa

½ cup sour cream

1 cup shredded lettuce

Directions:

In a bowl, put the coriander, garlic powder, salt, cumin, chili powder, and pepper. Mix well. Add the meat and lime juice. Stir and leave to marinate for 10 minutes. Add peppers and onion, and toss to combine.

Put half of the mixture in the cooking basket of the Air Fryer. Spray it with non-stick cooking spray.

Cook for 8 minutes at 4000F.

Reserve on a dish to cook the other mixture.

Put the tortillas in the cooking basket. Set the fryer to 190 degrees and cook for 3 minutes.

Divide the cooked meat as filling for the tortillas.

Serve with the ingredients for garnishing.

35. Honey Glazed Chicken Wings

Preparation Time: 10 minutes

Cooking Time: 20 minutes

Servings: 4

Nutrition:

Calories: 193

Fat: 11.1g

Carbs: 10.8g

Protein: 11g

Ingredients:

1 sliced onion

7 medium-sized chicken wings

Honey

For the marinade:

½ tsp. chopped ginger

1/8 tsp. pepper

1 tbsp. Chinese cooking wine

½ tbsp. soy sauce

½ tsp. chopped garlic

¼ tsp. sugar

½ tsp. five-spice powder

Directions:

Rinse the meat and pat them dry.

Mix all marinade ingredients in a bowl.

Add the meat to marinate for an hour.

Spread the onion slices on a pan. Lay the meat on top.

Put the rack inside the cooking basket and place the pan on top.

Cook for 10 minutes at 3500F.

Flip the meat and brush with honey. Cook for 5 more minutes. Flip and brush with honey.

Cook for 5 more minutes.

Enjoy.

36. Lamb Roast with Macadamia Crust

Preparation Time: 10 minutes

Cooking Time: 35 minutes

Servings: 6

Nutrition:

Calories: 215

Fat: 16.9g

Carbs: 3.4g

Protein: 13.7g

Ingredients:

1 ¾ pound rack of lamb

1 tbsp. olive oil

1 peeled garlic clove

Salt. Pepper

For the macadamia crust:

1 egg

3 oz. chopped macadamia nuts

1 tbsp. breadcrumbs

1 tbsp. chopped rosemary

Directions:

Prepare garlic oil.

Mix the olive oil and minced garlic in a bowl.

Brush the meat with garlic oil. Season with salt and pepper.

Put the chopped nuts, rosemary, and breadcrumbs in a bowl. Mix well.

Whisk the eggs in another bowl.

Dip the lamb into the egg mixture. Drain the excess liquid and cover with the macadamia crust. Arrange the coated meat in the cooking basket.

Cook for 30 minutes at 2200F.

Cook for 5 more minutes at 3900F.

Transfer into a plate and loosely cover with foil.

Leave for 10 minutes to rest before serving.

37. Black Bean Burger

Preparation Time: 5 minutes

Cooking Time: 35 minutes

Servings: 6

Nutrition:

Calories: 350

Fat: 2.6g

Carbs: 64.6g

Protein: 19.9g

Ingredients:

16 oz. black beans

1 1/3 cup rolled oats

¾ cup salsa

1 tbsp. soy sauce

½ tsp. chipotle chili powder

½ cup corn kernels

½ tsp. garlic powder

1¼ tsps. mild chili powder

Directions:

Put the oats in a food processor. Pulse up to 6 times or until partially chopped. Add the remaining ingredients, except the corn. Pulse until blended.

Transfer the bean mixture to a bowl. Add the corn and mix until combined. Chill for 15 minutes while covered.

Divide the bean mixture into 6 and form them into patties.

Arrange in the cooking basket lined with a perforated parchment paper. Lightly spray the patties with oil.

Cook for 15 minutes at 3750F.

38. Cheddar Bacon Croquettes

Preparation Time: 15 minutes

Cooking Time: 28 minutes

Servings: 4

Nutrition:

Calories: 962

Fat: 68.6g

Carbs: 32g

Protein: 53.1g

Ingredients:

For the breading:

2 eggs

1 cup all-purpose flour

1 cup seasoned breadcrumbs

4 tbsps. olive oil

For the filling:

1 lb. sharp cheddar cheese

1 lb. bacon slices

Directions:

Cut the cheese into 6 equal portions. Wrap each piece with 2 bacon slices. Trim excess fat. Chill for 5 minutes.

Mix the oil and breadcrumbs in a shallow bowl.

Dip each bacon wrapped cheese in the flour, cover with eggs and roll in breadcrumbs mixture. Arrange in the cooking basket.

Cook for 8 minutes at 3900F.

39. Steak with Spring Onion Salsa

Preparation Time: 5 minutes

Cooking Time: 12 minutes

Servings: 4

Nutrition:

Calories: 490

Protein: 63.73 g

Fat: 25.34 g

Carbs: 2.66 g

Ingredients:

2 lbs. steak

1 bunch chopped coriander leaves

2-3 sliced tomatoes

2 tsps. olive oil

1 tsp. black pepper

1 cup chopped spring onion

1 tsp. salt

Directions:

Pierce steak with a fork and season with salt and pepper. Drizzle with some olive oil.

Preheat Air Fryer at a temperature of 400°F (200°C).

Transfer steak into fryer basket and cook for 6 minutes.

After this time turn the side and cook for another 6 minutes or until nicely browned.

Slice steak with a sharp knife.

In a blender add spring onion, coriander, some salt, lime juice and green chili, blend until pureed.

Transfer steak on a platter with spring onion salsa.

Place tomatoes on a platter and drizzle some olive oil and sprinkle some black pepper on top.

Serve!

40. Stuffed Sweet Potatoes with Turkey

Preparation Time: 5 minutes

Cooking Time: 15 minutes

Servings: 4

Nutrition:

Calories: 190

Protein: 14.35 g

Fat: 7.99 g

Carbs: 15.7 g

Ingredients:

½ lb. turkey

2 medium sliced onion

1 chopped tomato

½ tsp. sea salt

2-3 minced garlic cloves

2 large halved sweet potatoes

½ tsp. smoked paprika

2 tbsps. olive oil

¼ tsp. cinnamon powder

Directions:

Heat half of olive oil in a pan and fry onions with garlic for 1-2 minutes.

Now add turkey pieces and fry until no longer pink.

Now add tomato, smoked paprika, salt. Fry for few minutes.

Add in cinnamon powder and mix, transfer into a bowl and set aside.

Now sprinkle some salt on sweet potatoes and drizzle olive oil.

Preheat your Air Fryer to a temperature of 400°F.

Place sweet potatoes into fryer basket and cook for 10 minutes.

Now remove from the fryer and scoop out some pulp of sweet potatoes and transfer it into turkey mixture, combine well.

Stuff sweet potatoes with turkey mixture and place into the fryer, cook for 5 minutes.

Serve!

41. Ground Beef and Rice Stuffed Bell Peppers

Preparation Time: 5 minutes

Cooking Time: 20 minutes

Servings: 4

Nutrition:

Calories: 446

Protein: 34.08 g

Fat: 28.03 g

Carbs: 22.86 g

Ingredients:

1 lb. ground beef

1 cup cooked rice

4 bell peppers

1 inch chopped ginger slice

1 small chopped onion

Salt. Pepper

1 tbsp. olive oil

1 tsp. garlic powder

Directions:

In a bowl add ground beef, rice, olive oil, ginger, salt, pepper, and onion, mix well.

Cut the stem of bell pepper and remove seeds.

Fill bell peppers with ground beef mixture.

Preheat Air Fryer to a temperature of 400°F (200°C).

Transfer bell peppers into fryer basket and cook for 20 minutes.

Serve!

42. Turmeric and Honey Chicken Drumsticks

Preparation Time: 5 minutes

Cooking Time: 20 minutes

Servings: 4

Nutrition:

Calories: 288

Protein: 30.88 g

Fat: 16.84 g

Carbs: 1.42 g

Ingredients:

1½ pound chicken drumsticks

1 tsp. ginger paste

¼ tsp. garlic paste

1 tsp. cooking oil

½ tsp. chili powder

¼ tsp. turmeric powder

¼ tsp. salt

¼ tsp. cinnamon powder

2 tbsps. lime juice

Directions:

Preheat Air Fryer at a temperature of 370°F (190°C).

In a large bowl add lime juice, cooking oil, salt, chili powder, turmeric powder, cinnamon powder, and ginger garlic paste, mix well.

Now add in drumsticks and toss to combine.

Place drumsticks into Air Fryer basket and let cook for 20 minutes.

After halftime turn the sides and cook until nicely golden.

Serve!

43. Jamaican Jerk Pork

Preparation Time: 10 minutes

Cooking Time: 20 minutes

Servings: 4

Nutrition:

Calories: 338

Fat: 12g

Carbs: 1.1g

Protein: 53g

Ingredients:

1.5 lbs. chopped pork butt

¼ cup jerk paste

Directions:

Rub meat with the jerk paste.

Chill for at least 4 hours to marinate.

Leave at room temperature for 20 minutes before cooking.

Spray the bottom part of the cooking basket with oil before putting the marinated meat.

Cook for 20 minutes at 3900F. Flip the meat halfway through the cooking process.

Transfer to a platter and leave for 10 minutes to rest before serving.

44. Fried Meatballs in Tomato Sauce

Preparation Time: 12 minutes

Cooking Time: 25 minutes

Servings: 4

Nutrition:

Calories: 436

Fat: 14g

Carbs: 10.8g

Protein: 63.6g

Ingredients:

1 egg

½ tbsp. chopped thyme leaves

¾ lb. ground beef

1 chopped onion

1 tbsp. chopped parsley

10 oz. tomato sauce

Pepper. Salt

3 tbsps. breadcrumbs

Directions:

Combine all the ingredients in a bowl.

Form 12 small balls from the mixture using your hands.

Arrange them in the cooking basket.

Cook for 8 minutes at 3900F. Transfer the meatballs to an oven dish. Drizzle with tomato sauce on top.

Place the oven dish in the cooking basket and cook for 5 minutes at 330 degrees.

45. Garlic Herb Butter Steak

Preparation Time: 15 minutes

Cooking Time: 17 minutes

Servings: 2

Nutrition:

Calories: 1905

Fat: 89g

Carbs: 1.7g

Protein: 250g

Ingredients:

2- 8oz. rib eye steak

1 stick unsalted butter

1 tsp. Worcestershire sauce

2 tsps. garlic minced

2 tbsps. chopped fresh parsley

Garlic butter

Olive oil

Cracked Black pepper

½ tsp. salt

Directions:

Prepare the garlic butter. Put Worcestershire sauce, garlic, parsley, and butter in a bowl. Mix well. Season with salt. Transfer to a parchment paper and roll like a log. Chill until ready to cook.

Rub all sides of the steak with olive oil. Season with black pepper and salt.

Grease the fryer's cooking basket before placing the meat. Cook for 12 minutes in a preheated Air Fryer at 400 degrees. Flip the meat halfway through the cooking process.

Set on a plate to rest for 5 minutes. Add garlic butter on top before serving.

46. Air Fryer Meatloaf

Preparation Time: 5 minutes

Cooking Time: 45 minutes

Servings: 8

Nutrition:

Calories: 290

Fat: 8.9g

Carbs: 10.7g

Protein: 36g

Ingredients:

2 lbs. ground beef

¼ cup beef broth

2 eggs

½ cup chopped mushrooms

1 cup fresh soft bread crumbs

1 tbsp. Dijon style mustard

½ tsp. kosher salt

1 tbsp. Worcestershire sauce

3 tbsps. ketchup

2 garlic cloves

½ cup shredded carrots

For the glaze

¼ cup brown sugar

2 tsps. Dijon mustard

½ cup ketchup

Directions:

Mix beef broth and breadcrumbs in a bowl. Set aside.

Put garlic, onions, carrots, and mushrooms in a food processor. Process until finely chopped. Transfer to a bowl. Add meat, Worcestershire sauce, Dijon mustard, ketchup, and the broth and breadcrumb mixture. Mix well. Season with salt. Use your hands to combine all ingredients and shape the mixture into a loaf.

Place the meatloaf in a greased cooking basket. Cook for 45 minutes in a preheated Air Fryer at 390 degrees.

Prepare the glaze. Combine all ingredients for the glaze in a bowl. Open the cooking basket of the Air Fryer 5 minutes before the cooking process is done. Brush glaze all over the meatloaf and continue cooking.

Transfer meatloaf to a plate.

Let it rest for 10 minutes then serve.

47. Cod Fish Nuggets

Preparation Time: 10 minutes

Cooking Time: 15 minutes

Servings: 4

Nutrition:

Calories: 404

Fat: 11.6g

Carbs: 38.6g

Protein: 34.6g

Ingredients:

1 lb. sliced cod

For the breading:

1 cup all-purpose flour

2 eggs

A pinch of salt

2 tbsps. olive oil

¾ cup breadcrumbs

Directions:

Put olive oil, salt, and panko breadcrumbs in a food processor. Process until fine. Transfer mixture to a bowl.

Put the flour and the beaten eggs in separate bowls.

Coat each cod strip with flour, then in the eggs and finally coat with breadcrumbs. Press the coating to make it stick.

Arrange the coated cod pieces in the cooking basket.

Cook for 10 minutes at 3900F.

48. Air Fryer Bacon Wrapped Shrimp

Preparation Time: 5 minutes

Cooking Time: 27 minutes

Servings: 4

Nutrition:

Calories: 436

Fat: 41.01g

Carbs: 0.86g

Protein: 15.64g

Ingredients:

16 pieces of peeled tiger shrimp

16 thin slices of bacon

Directions:

Cover each shrimp with a slice of bacon.

Put all the finished pieces in tray and chill for 20 minutes.

Arrange the bacon wrapped shrimp in the cooking basket.

Cook for 7 minutes at 3900F.

Set on a lined plate with paper towels to drain before serving.

49. Salmon with Dill Sauce

Preparation Time: 15 minutes

Cooking Time: 30 minutes

Servings: 4

Nutrition:

Calories: 348

Fat: 18.97g

Carbs: 5.29g

Protein: 37.694g

Ingredients:

4 6-oz. pieces of salmon

2 tsps. olive oil

Salt

For the dill sauce:

½ cup sour cream

½ cup non-fat Greek yogurt

2 tbsps. chopped dill

A pinch of salt

Directions:

Rub each salmon piece with olive oil. Season with salt. Put them in the cooking basket. Cook for 30 minutes at 2700F.

To make the sauce, set all the sauce ingredients in a bowl. Mix well.

Serve the fish with the sauce.

Top with chopped dill.

50. Coconut Spiced Shrimp

Preparation Time: 22 minutes

Cooking Time: 6 minutes

Servings: 4

Nutrition:

Calories: 239

Fat: 8.67g

Carbs: 22.05g

Protein: 16.69g

Ingredients:

½ lb. peeled jumbo shrimp

2 eggs

1/3 cup panko breadcrumbs

½ cup cornstarch

½ cup sweetened coconut flakes

1 tbsp. water

½ tsp. salt

Directions:

Beat egg and water in a shallow baking dish. Mix the coconut flakes, breadcrumbs, and salt in another baking dish.

Put the cornstarch and shrimp in a zip bag. Shake until evenly coated.

Pass each piece of shrimp in the egg mixture and coat with the breadcrumb mixture.

Arrange 6 coated shrimp in the cooking basket of the Air Fryer at a time.

Set to 400 degrees and cook for 6 minutes.

Transfer to a platter and cook the rest of the shrimp.

51. Teriyaki Halibut Steak

Preparation Time: 40 minutes

Cooking Time: 12 minutes

Servings: 3

Nutrition:

Calories: 374

Fat: 21.22g

Carbs: 18.12g

Protein: 27.82g

Ingredients:

1 lb. halibut steak

For the marinade:

¼ tsp. crushed red pepper flakes

¼ tsp. ground ginger

¼ cup sugar

¼ cup mirin

¼ cup orange juice

2 tbsps. lime juice

1 smashed garlic clove

2/3 cup low-sodium soy sauce

Directions:

Set all the marinade ingredients in a pan over medium flame.

Bring to a boil while stirring often. Set aside to cool.

Transfer half of the marinade in a Ziploc bag. Add the halibut steak and seal.
Chill for at least half an hour.

Place the marinated halibut steak in the cooking basket. Cook for 12 minutes
at 3900F.

Brush the remaining marinade over the steak before serving.

52. Air Fryer Crab Cakes

Preparation Time: 42 minutes

Cooking Time: 10 minutes

Servings: 4

Nutrition:

Calories: 303

Fat: 15.61g

Carbs: 28.39g

Protein: 13.22g

Ingredients:

1 egg

500 grams thawed frozen crab meat

1 tbsp. mayonnaise

3 stalks chopped spring onions

6 pieces crushed butter crackers

½ tsp. garlic powder

Black pepper

1 tbsp. corn flour

1 chopped yellow onion

½ tsp. salt

Directions:

Boil the water then remove from heat.

Soak the crab meat in boiling water for a couple of seconds. Drain excess moist and place on a plate lined with paper towels.

Put the crab meat in a bowl. Add the rest of the ingredients. Mix until combined.

Mold mixture into your desired shapes and sizes using your hands.

Arrange the crab cakes in the cooking basket. Cook for 10 minutes at 3500F.

53. Italian Chicken Tenders

Preparation Time: 15 minutes

Cooking Time: 10 minutes

Servings: 4

Nutrition:

Calories: 441

Fat: 25.4 g

Carbs: 8.3 g

Protein: 42.4 g

Ingredients:

Chicken tenders, 1 ½ lbs.

Eggs, 2.

Fine almond flour, 1 cup

Garlic powder, ½ tsp.

Italian seasoning, 1 tsp.

Fine sea salt, 1 tsp.

Ground black pepper, ½ tsp.

Onion powder, ½ tsp.

Avocado oil spray

Ground flaxseed, 2 tbsps.

Paprika, 1 tsp.

Directions:

Let your air fryer preheat to 4000 F.

Using a paper towel, dry the chicken then season it with pepper and salt.

Whisk egg in a suitable bowl and keep it aside.

Mix almond flour, seasonings, and flaxseed in a shallow bowl.

Pass the chicken in the egg then dredge it through the dry flour mixture.

Shake off the excess then place it in the air fryer basket.

Spray the tenders with avocado oil and return the basket to the fryer.

Cook them for 5 minutes on Air Fry Mode.

Then flip the pieces and return them to the air fryer for another 5 minutes.

Serve warm.

54. Salmon Cakes

Preparation Time: 15 minutes

Cooking Time: 16 minutes

Servings: 4

Nutrition:

Calories: 251

Fat: 15.3 g

Carbs: 3 g

Protein: 25 g

Ingredients:

Fresh Atlantic salmon, 1 lb.

Brown eggs, 2.

Diced cilantro, ¼ cup

Tapioca starch, ¼ cup

Coconut flakes, ½ cup

Melted coconut oil.

Yellow curry powder, 1 ½ tsp.

Tapioca starch, 4 tsp.

Sea salt, ½ tsp.

Mashed avocado, ¼ cup

For the greens:

Sea salt, ¼ tsp.

Tightly packed arugula and spinach mix, 6 cup

Melted organic coconut oil, 2 tsp.

Directions:

Remove the fish skin and dice the flesh. Place it a large bowl.

Add cilantro, avocado, salt, and curry powder and mix gently.

Add tapioca starch and mix well again.

Make 8 salmon patties out of this mixture, about a half inch thick.

Place them in a baking sheet lined with wax paper and freeze them for 20 minutes.

Meanwhile, preheat air fryer at 4000 F in 10 minutes.

Place ¼ cup tapioca starch and coconut flakes on a flat plate.

Whisk eggs then dip the frozen patties in them then coat them in the starch and flakes.

Place the patties in the air fryer basket and spray them with cooking oil.

Cook them for 15 minutes in the air fryer on Air Fry Mode.

Sauté arugula with spinach in coconut oil in a pan for 1 minute.

Serve the patties with sautéed greens mixture.

55. Ranch Cauliflower Patties

Preparation Time: 15 minutes

Cooking Time: 20 minutes

Servings: 2

Nutrition:

Calories: 201

Fat: 7.8 g

Carbs: 4.1 g

Protein: 7.8 g

Ingredients:

Grated cauliflower florets, 2 cup

Chopped green onion, 1.

Packed cilantro, 1 cup

Sunflower seeds, ¼ cup

Minced garlic, 1 tsp.

Chilli powder, ½ tsp.

Cornstarch, 2 tbsps.

Cumin, ¼ tsp.

Pepper, ¼ tsp.

Organic ranch seasoning mix, 2 tbsps.

Ground flaxseed, ¼ cup

Kosher salt, ¼ tsp.

Any dipping sauce.

Directions:

Let your oven preheat to 4000 F. Grease the basket with cooking oil.

Toss all the vegetables in a food processor and grind them together.

Add flaxseed, sunflower seeds, all the seasoning, cornstarch, and cilantro.

Stir thoroughly until it forms a thick batter.

Make 1.5-inch thick patties out of it.

Place 4 patties in the air fryer basket then return the basket to the air fryer.

Cook them for 20 minutes on Air Fry Mode, flipping them halfway through.

Cook the remaining patties using the same steps.

Serve.

56. Parmesan Crusted Pork Chops

Preparation Time: 10

Cooking Time: 15 minutes

Servings: 4

Nutrition:

Calories: 381

Carbs: 5g

Protein: 42g

Fat: 24g

Ingredients:

Centre-cut boneless pork chops, 4.

Large free-range eggs, 2.

Pork rind crumbs, 1 cup

Pepper, ¼ tsp.

Onion powder, ½ tsp.

Chilli powder, ¼ tsp.

Smoked paprika, 1 tsp.

Salt, ½ tsp.

Grated parmesan cheese, 3 tbsps.

Directions:

Preheat your air fryer to 400°F.

Place the pork chops onto a flat surface and season with salt and pepper.

Grab your food processor and add the pork rinds. Blend until they form crumbs.

Place the crumbs into a large bowl with the seasoning and stir well to combine.

Grab a medium bowl and add the beaten eggs.

Take each pork chop and dip into the egg mixture, allowing any excess to drip off then pop into the crumbs.

Cook for 15 minutes until delicious!

Serve and enjoy.

57. Honey Mustard Pork Chops

Preparation Time: 10 minutes

Cooking Time: 12 minutes

Servings: 4

Nutrition:

Calories: 138

Carbs: 9g

Protein: 5g

Fat: 14g

Ingredients:

Pork chops, 4.

Minced garlic, 2 tbsps.

Mustard, 4 tbsps.

Salt, 1 tsp.

Honey, 2 tbsps.

Pepper, 1 tsp.

Directions:

Preheat the air fryer to 350°F.

Grab a large bowl and combine the mustard, honey, garlic, salt and pepper. Stir well.

Place the pork chops into the mustard mixture and stir well to coat.

Spray the air fryer basket then place the chops inside.

Air fry for 12 minutes until cooked, flipping often.

Serve and enjoy.

58. Coffee & Spice Ribeye Steak

Preparation Time: 20 minutes

Cooking Time: 10 minutes

Servings: 2

Nutrition:

Calories: 495

Carbs: 5g

Protein: 46g

Fat: 32g

Ingredients:

Ribeye steak, 1 lb.

Chipotle powder, ¼ tsp.

Sweetener, 1 tsp.

Chilli powder, ¼ tsp.

Onion powder, ¼ tsp.

Coriander, 1/8 tsp.

Black pepper, ½ tsp.

Ground coffee, ½ tsp.

Paprika, ¼ tsp.

Cocoa powder, 1/8 tsp.

Coarse sea salt, 1 ½ tsp.

Garlic powder, ¼ tsp.

Directions:

Preheat your air fryer to 390°F.

Meanwhile, grab a medium bowl, add all the spices and stir well to combine.

Grab a flat dish and sprinkle with plenty of the spice mixture.

Pop the steaks into the spice mixture and stir well, pushing the spice mixture into the flesh.

Leave to rest for 10-20 minutes.

Spray your air fryer with some oil then place the steaks inside.

Cook for 10 minutes.

When fully cooked, allow to rest for 5 minutes before serving.

59. Beef Satay

Preparation Time: 10 minutes

Cooking Time: 10 minutes

Servings: 4

Nutrition:

Calories: 252

Carbs: 5g

Protein: 14g

Fat: 24g

Ingredients:

Thinly sliced beef flank steak, 1 lb.

For the marinade:

Chopped cilantro, ¼ cup.

Minced ginger, 1 tbsp.

Sriracha sauce, 1 tsp.

Ground coriander, 1 tsp.

Fish sauce, 1 tbsp.

Minced garlic, 1 tbsp.

Sugar, 1 tbsp.

Oil, 2 tbsps.

Soy sauce, 1 tbsp.

For serving:

Chopped roasted peanuts, ¼ cup

Directions:

Grab a medium bowl and add the marinade ingredients. Stir well.

Pop the beef into the marinade and stir well.

Leave in the fridge for 30 minutes to marinate.

Preheat your air fryer to 400°F.

Place the beef strips into the air fryer and cook for 10 minutes, turning midway through cooking.

Top with the peanuts plus extra cilantro then enjoy

60. Beef Lasagna

Preparation Time: 15 minutes

Cooking Time: 20 minutes

Servings: 4

Nutrition:

Calories: 838

Carbs: 10g

Protein: 62g

Fat: 65g

Ingredients:

For the meat layer:

Ground beef, 1 lb.

Diced celery, ¼ cup

Diced red onion, ¼ cup

Minced garlic, ½ tsp.

Prepared marinara sauce, 1 cup

Olive oil

Pepper. Salt

For the cheese layer:

Large free-range eggs, 2.

Dried Italian seasoning, 1 tsp.

Divided shredded cheese, 1 cup

Minced garlic, ½ tsp.

Ricotta cheese, 8 oz.

Grated parmesan cheese, ½ cup

For the topping:

Grated mozzarella.

Directions:

Preheat your air fryer to 375°F and grease a pan that will fit into your air fryer.

Take a large bowl and add the ingredients for the meat layer. Stir well to combine.

Place the meat into the pan, spreading evenly.

Pop into the air fryer and cook for 10 minutes.

Meanwhile, take another bowl and add the cheese layer ingredients. Stir well.

Get the pan from the air fryer and add the cheese mixture.

Spread well then top with the mozzarella. Pop into the air fryer again.

Cook for 10 minutes then remove and leave to rest for 5 minutes.

Serve and enjoy.

61. BBQ Chicken Wings

Preparation Time: 10 minutes

Cooking Time: 15 minutes

Servings: 4

Nutrition:

Calories: 330

Carbs: 35g

Protein: 2g

Fat: 18g

Ingredients:

Chicken wings, 1 ¾ lb.

Olive oil, 1 tsp.

Garlic powder, 1 tsp.

Barbecue sauce, 2 tbsps.

Smoked paprika, 1 tsp.

Salt. Pepper.

Directions:

Preheat the air fryer to 360°F.

Grab a large bowl and add the garlic powder, paprika, salt and pepper. Stir well.

Add the oil and stir again, then place the chicken wings inside. Stir again to coat.

Set the chicken into the air fryer basket to cook for 12 minutes, flipping often.

Remove from the fryer and place back into the bowl.

Add the barbeque sauce, stir well then place back into the air fryer.

Allow to cook for 3 minutes then serve.

62. Buffalo Chicken Legs

Preparation Time: 5 minutes

Cooking Time: 25 minutes

Servings: 4

Nutrition:

Calories: 476

Carbs: 0g

Protein: 30g

Fat: 50g

Ingredients:

Skinless chicken drumsticks, 2 lb.

Hot sauce, ¼ cup

Melted butter, 2 tbsps.

Directions:

Preheat the air fryer to 400°F.

Spray the air fryer with oil then cook the drumsticks for 20 minutes, flipping midway through cooking.

Place the butter and hot sauce in a bowl, stir well then add the cooked chicken. Stir well to coat then return to the air fryer.

Leave to cook until crispy, about 5 minutes.

Serve and enjoy!

63. Chicken Coconut Meatballs

Preparation Time: 10 minutes

Cooking Time: 10 minutes

Servings: 4

Nutrition:

Calories: 223

Carbs: 3g

Protein: 20g

Fat: 14g

Ingredients:

Ground chicken, 1 lb.

Unsweetened shredded coconut, ¼ cup

Hoisin sauce, 1 tbsp.

Finely chopped green onions, 2.

Chopped cilantro, ½ cup

Sriracha, 1 tbsp.

Soy sauce, 1 tbsp.

Sesame oil, 1 tbsp.

Pepper. Salt.

Directions:

Preheat your air fryer to 350°F.

Grab a large bowl and add all the ingredients. Stir well together.

Using your hands, shape into meatballs and pop into the air fryer.

Cook for 10 minutes, turning midway through cooking.

Serve and enjoy.

64. Jalapeno Popper Stuffed Chicken Breast

Preparation Time: 10 minutes

Cooking Time: 20 minutes

Servings: 4

Nutrition:

Calories: 654

Carbs: 2g

Protein: 62g

Fat: 42g

Ingredients:

Butterflied chicken breasts, 16 oz.

Cheddar cheese, 4 oz.

Jalapeños, 2.

Stripped bacon, 8.

Cream cheese, 4 oz.

Directions:

Preheat your air fryer to 370°F.

Place the chicken onto a flat surface and spread the inside with cream cheese.

Add half the jalapenos to each chicken breast and top with cheddar cheese.

Close the chicken then wrap with two slices of bacon.

Cook for 20 minutes, turning often.

Serve and enjoy.

65. Spicy Mexican Chicken Burgers

Preparation Time: 10 minutes

Cooking Time: 30 minutes

Servings: 4

Nutrition:

Calories: 240

Carbs: 14g

Protein: 32g

Fat: 7g

Ingredients:

Skinless and deboned chicken breasts, 4.

Jalapeno pepper, 1.

Free-range egg, 1.

Small cauliflower, 1.

Dried thyme, 1 tbsp.

Mustard powder, 1 tbsp.

Cayenne pepper, 1 tsp.

Salt.

Oregano, 1 tbsp.

Smoked paprika, 3 tbsps.

Pepper.

Directions:

Preheat the air fryer to 350°F.

Grab your blender and add the cauliflower and the seasoning. Whizz until it looks like breadcrumbs.

Place ¾ of breadcrumbs into a bowl and the remaining ¼ into another bowl.

Add the egg to the ¼ portion and stir well. Pop to one side.

Take your blender again and add the chicken and ¼ of cauliflower and seasoning mixture. Season well then whizz again.

Using your hands, form into patties.

Dip the patties into the beaten egg mixture then toss in the remaining seasoned cauliflower.

Cook in the air fryer for 30 minutes, turning halfway through.

Serve and enjoy.

66. Turkey Breast

Preparation Time: 10 minutes

Cooking Time: 40 minutes

Servings: 8

Nutrition:

Calories: 226

Carbs: 0g

Protein: 33g

Fat: 10g

Ingredients:

Deboned turkey breast, 4 lb.

Kosher, 2 tsps.

Olive oil, 1 tbsp.

Dry turkey seasoning, ½ tbsps.

Directions:

Preheat your air fryer to 350°F

Rub the turkey breast with olive oil over the flesh.

Season with salt and pepper then place into the air fryer.

Cook for 40 minutes.

Leave to rest once cooked for 10 minutes

Serve and enjoy.

Chapter 3.Dinner recipes

67. BBQ Pork Bowls

Preparation time: 5 minutes

Cooking time: 20 minutes

Servings: 4

Ingredients:

1/3 cup bbq sauce

2 tablespoons honey

1 pound pork stew meat, cubed

1 red onion, chopped

1 zucchini, cubed

2 tablespoons olive oil

2 tomatoes, cubed

Directions:

Heat up the air fryer with the oil at 380 degrees F, add the onion and the meat and brown for 5 minutes.

Add the rest of the ingredients, toss, cook for 15 minutes more, divide everything into bowls and serve.

Nutrition: calories 393, fat 18.3, fiber 2, carbs 22.8, protein 34.7

68. Turkey Pie

Preparation time: 10 minutes

Cooking time: 20 minutes

Servings: 4

Ingredients:

1 pound turkey breast, boneless, skinless and cubed

1 red onion, chopped

2 tomatoes, cubed

1 cup mushrooms, chopped

1 teaspoon balsamic vinegar

Salt and black pepper to the taste

1 teaspoon coriander, chopped

1 teaspoon onion powder

½ teaspoon garlic powder

1 tablespoon white flour

1 tablespoon almond milk

2 puff pastry sheets

2 tablespoons avocado oil

Directions:

Heat up a pan with half of the oil over medium heat, add the meat, onion, mushrooms and the other ingredients except the puff pastry, toss, cook for 5 minutes and take off the heat.

Place 1 puff pastry sheet on the bottom of your air fryer's pan, add the turkey mix, top with the other puff pastry sheet, brush with the remaining oil, place the pan in the fryer, cook at 370 degrees F for 15 minutes, slice and serve for lunch.

Nutrition: calories 172, fat 3.9, fiber 2.6, carbs 13.1, protein 21.3

69. Parmesan Chicken Mix

Preparation time: 10 minutes

Cooking time: 20 minutes

Servings: 4

Ingredients:

1 tablespoon olive oil

1 yellow onion, sliced

1 pound chicken breasts, skinless, boneless and roughly cubed

Salt and black pepper to the taste

1 tablespoon balsamic vinegar

1 cup cherry tomatoes, halved

1 cup eggplant, cubed

1 cup parmesan cheese, grated

½ cup tomato sauce

1 tablespoon cilantro, chopped

Directions:

Preheat your air fryer with the oil at 380 degrees F, add the chicken and the onion and cook for 5 minutes.

Add the rest of the ingredients, toss, cook for 15 minutes more, divide into bowls and serve for lunch.

Nutrition: calories 278, fat 12.1, fiber 2.3, carbs 7.2, protein 34.1

70. Pork and Potatoes Mix

Preparation time: 10 minutes

Cooking time: 20 minutes

Servings: 4

Ingredients:

2 pounds pork stew meat, cubed

4 gold potatoes, peeled and cut into wedges

2 tablespoons olive oil

2 red onions, sliced

Salt and black pepper to the taste

1 teaspoon rosemary, dried

1 teaspoon garam masala

1 teaspoon oregano, dried

1 tablespoon chives, chopped

Directions:

Heat up the air fryer with the oil at 370 degrees F, add the onion and the meat and brown for 5 minutes.

Add the potatoes and the other ingredients, toss, and cook for 15 minutes more.

Divide the mix between plates and serve for lunch.

Nutrition: calories 565, fat 29.1, fiber 1.5, carbs 5.6, protein 67.1

71. Lemony Chicken Wings

Preparation time: 10 minutes

Cooking time: 35 minutes

Servings: 4

Ingredients:

2 pounds chicken wings

3 tablespoons avocado oil

1 tablespoon sweet paprika

A pinch of salt and black pepper

1 tablespoon lemon juice

Directions:

In a bowl, combine the chicken wings with the oil and the other ingredients, toss well, put them in your air fryer's basket and cook them at 360 degrees F for 35 minutes shaking the fryer from time to time.

Divide the chicken wings between plates and serve for lunch with a side salad.

Nutrition: calories 451, fat 18.4, fiber 1.1, carbs 1.7, protein 66

72. Sausage Pan

Preparation time: 10 minutes

Cooking time: 15 minutes

Servings: 4

Ingredients:

1 pound pork sausages, sliced

1 yellow onion, chopped

2 gold potatoes, peeled and cubed

2 tablespoons olive oil

½ cup tomato sauce

A pinch of salt and black pepper

2 tablespoons parmesan cheese, grated

Directions:

Heat up the air fryer with the oil at 370 degrees F, add the sausage and the onion and cook for 5 minutes.

Add the other ingredients, toss, cook for 10 minutes more, divide between plates and serve for lunch.

Nutrition: calories 463, fat 38.3, fiber 1.1, carbs 4.2, protein 22.7

73. Lentils Stew

Preparation time: 5 minutes

Cooking time: 20 minutes

Servings: 4

Ingredients:

1 cup canned yellow lentils, drained

1 cup canned red lentils, drained

1 tablespoon ginger, grated

1 red onion, chopped

2 tablespoons olive oil

1 cup veggie stock

½ teaspoon turmeric powder

1 teaspoon garam masala

Salt and black pepper to the taste

½ cup cilantro, chopped

1 cup baby spinach, chopped

4 garlic cloves, minced

½ cup tomato passata

Directions:

Heat up your air fryer with the oil at 370 degrees F, add the ginger, onion ,turmeric and garam masala and cook for 5 minutes.

Add the lentils and the other ingredients, toss and cook everything for 15 minutes more.

Divide the stew into bowls and serve for lunch.

Nutrition: calories 309, fat 7.9, fiber 19.7, carbs 43.6, protein 17.7

74. Ground Beef and Tomatoes

Preparation time: 5 minutes

Cooking time: 20 minutes

Servings: 4

Ingredients:

1 pound lean beef, ground

2 tablespoons olive oil

2 cups tomatoes, cubed

2 spring onions, chopped

1 red onion, chopped

2 garlic cloves, minced

1 tablespoon basil, chopped

Salt and black pepper to the taste

½ cup tomato sauce

Directions:

Heat up the air fryer with the oil at 360 degrees F, add the onion and spring onion and cook for 2 minutes.

Add the meat and cook for 3 minutes more.

Add the rest of the ingredients, toss, and cook for 15 minutes.

Divide everything into bowls and serve for lunch.

Nutrition: calories 310, fat 14.4, fiber 2.4, carbs 8.8, protein 36.2

75. Beef Meatballs Bowls

Preparation time: 10 minutes

Cooking time: 20 minutes

Servings: 4

Ingredients:

1 pound beef, minced

½ cup tomato sauce

1 yellow onion, chopped

2 garlic cloves, minced

1 egg, whisked

1 tablespoon bread crumbs

2 tablespoons olive oil

1 cup baby spinach

1 cup cherry tomatoes, halved

1 tablespoon oregano, chopped

Salt and black pepper to the taste

Directions:

In a bowl, combine the beef with the onion, garlic, the egg, bread crumbs, salt and pepper stir and shape medium meatballs out of this mixture.

Heat up your air fryer with the oil at 375 degrees F, add the meatballs, and cook them for 14 minutes flipping them halfway.

Add the tomato sauce and the other ingredients, toss gently, cook for 6 minutes more, divide into bowls and serve.

Nutrition: calories 280, fat 9, fiber 6, carbs 16, protein 15

76. Balsamic Cod Mix

Preparation time: 10 minutes

Cooking time: 12 minutes

Servings: 4

Ingredients:

4 cod fillets, boneless and skinless

1 tablespoon balsamic vinegar

2 tablespoons olive oil

Salt and black pepper to the taste

2 tablespoons walnuts, chopped

2 teaspoons coriander, ground

1 teaspoon rosemary, dried

Directions:

Put the fish in your air fryer's basket, add the vinegar and the other ingredients except the walnuts and cook at 400 degrees F for 12 minutes flipping the fish halfway.

Divide the fish between plates, sprinkle the walnuts on top and serve for lunch.

Nutrition: calories 240, fat 4, fiber 2, carbs 15, protein 12

77. Maple Chicken

Preparation time: 10 minutes

Cooking time: 30 minutes

Servings: 4

Ingredients:

1 pound chicken breast, skinless, boneless and sliced

1 tablespoon olive oil

½ teaspoon sweet paprika

1 teaspoon rosemary, dried

Salt and black pepper to the taste

2 tablespoons maple syrup

Directions:

In a bowl, combine the chicken breast slices with the oil, paprika and the other ingredients and toss well.

Put the chicken slices in your air fryer's basket and cook at 370 degrees F for 30 minutes, flipping the slices halfway.

Divide between plates and serve.

Nutrition: calories 230, fat 13, fiber 3, carbs 16, protein 11

78. Salmon Meatballs

Preparation time: 10 minutes

Cooking time: 12 minutes

Servings: 4

Ingredients:

2 tablespoons cilantro, minced

1 pound salmon fillets, boneless, skinless and minced

1 red onion, chopped

1 egg

Salt and black pepper to the taste

2 garlic cloves, minced

½ teaspoon turmeric powder

¼ cup almond flour

Cooking spray

Directions:

In a bowl, combine the salmon with the cilantro and the other ingredients except the cooking spray, stir well and shape medium meatballs out of this mix.

Place the meatballs in your air fryer's basket, grease them with the cooking spray, cook at 320 degrees F for 12 minutes shaking halfway, divide between plates and serve for lunch.

Nutrition: calories 230, fat 9, fiber 3, carbs 10, protein 15

79. Turkey Stew

Preparation time: 10 minutes

Cooking time: 20 minutes

Servings: 4

Ingredients:

2 pounds turkey breast, skinless, boneless and cubed

2 tablespoons olive oil

1 carrot, sliced

1 yellow onion, chopped

2 garlic cloves, minced

1 teaspoon rosemary, dried

Salt and black pepper to the taste

2 cups chicken stock

½ teaspoon cumin, ground

A handful cilantro, chopped

Directions:

In your air fryer's pan, combine the turkey with the oil, carrot and the other ingredients, toss and cook at 380 degrees F for 20 minutes.

Divide into bowls and serve right away.

Nutrition: calories 250, fat 8, fiber 1, carbs 20, protein 17

80. Shrimp Stew

Preparation time: 10 minutes

Cooking time: 15 minutes

Servings: 4

Ingredients:

1 pound shrimp, peeled and deveined

3 scallions, chopped

2 tablespoons olive oil

1 cup chicken stock

Salt and black pepper to the taste

2 garlic cloves, minced

1 teaspoon chili powder

1 zucchini, cubed

½ cup cherry tomatoes, halved

1 tablespoon cilantro, chopped

Directions:

Heat up the air fryer with the oil at 350 degrees F, add the scallions, garlic and chili powder and cook for 3 minutes.

Add the shrimp and the other ingredients, toss, cook for 12 minutes more, divide into bowls and serve for lunch.

Nutrition: calories 270, fat 7, fiber 4, carbs 15, protein 6

81. Cheesy Chicken and Zucchini

Preparation time: 5 minutes

Cooking time: 20 minutes

Servings: 4

Ingredients:

1 pound chicken breast, skinless, boneless and cubed

2 tablespoons olive oil

2 zucchinis, roughly cubed

4 scallions, chopped

1 teaspoon chili powder

1 teaspoon coriander, ground

1 tablespoon cilantro, chopped

¼ cup cheddar cheese, grated

Directions:

Heat up the air fryer with the oil at 370 degrees F, add the scallions, meat and chili powder and brown for 5 minutes.

Add the other ingredients, toss and cook for 15 minutes more.

Divide the mix into bowls and serve for lunch.

Nutrition: calories 260, fat 12, fiber 4, carbs 14, protein 11

82. Shrimp Curry

Preparation time: 10 minutes

Cooking time: 12 minutes

Servings: 4

Ingredients:

1 pound shrimp, peeled and deveined

1 yellow onion, chopped

2 tablespoons olive oil

2 teaspoons yellow curry paste

½ teaspoon turmeric powder

1 cup kale, torn

½ cup heavy cream

2 tablespoons cilantro, chopped

2 teaspoons ginger, grated

Salt and black pepper to the taste

Directions:

Heat up the air fryer with the oil at 360 degrees F, add the onion, curry paste and turmeric and cook for 2 minutes.

Add the shrimp and the other ingredients, cook everything for 10 minutes, divide into bowls and serve.

Nutrition: calories 260, fat 8, fiber 3, carbs 13, protein 9

83. Cream Cheese Chicken

Preparation time: 10 minutes

Cooking time: 25 minutes

Servings: 4

Ingredients:

2 tablespoons butter, melted

1 cup cream cheese, soft

1 pound chicken breast, skinless, boneless and cubed

2 teaspoons curry powder

4 scallions, chopped

¼ cup cilantro, chopped

Salt and black pepper to the taste

Directions:

In your air fryer's pan, combine the chicken with the cream cheese, the butter and the other ingredients, toss and cook at 350 degrees F for 25 minutes.

Divide between plates and serve for lunch.

Nutrition: calories 280, fat 10, fiber 2, carbs 24, protein 15

84. Italian Potato Stew

Preparation time: 5 minutes

Cooking time: 25 minutes

Servings: 4

Ingredients:

1 pound gold potatoes, peeled and cut into medium wedges

1 red onion, chopped

1 carrot, peeled and sliced

Salt and black pepper to the taste

1 tablespoon olive oil

1 and ½ teaspoon sweet paprika

½ cup tomato sauce

½ teaspoon Italian seasoning

1 tablespoon dill, chopped

Directions:

Heat up the air fryer with the oil at 370 degrees F, add the onion, paprika and Italian seasoning and cook for 5 minutes.

Add the potatoes and the other ingredients and cook everything for 20 minutes more.

Divide the stew into bowls and serve for lunch.

Nutrition: calories 290, fat 8, fiber 2, carbs 15, protein 7

85. Pork and Cabbage Stew

Preparation time: 10 minutes

Cooking time: 25 minutes

Servings: 4

Ingredients:

1 pound pork stew meat, cubed

1 yellow onion, chopped

1 cup tomato sauce

1 cup beef stock

1 green bell pepper, cut into strips

1 carrot, peeled and sliced

1 tablespoon olive oil

2 cups green cabbage, shredded

2 garlic cloves, minced

Salt and black pepper to the taste

1 tablespoon rosemary, dried

Directions:

In your air fryer's pan, combine the pork with the onion, stock, and the other ingredients, toss and cook at 370 degrees F for 25 minutes.

Divide into bowls and serve for lunch.

Nutrition: calories 262, fat 9, fiber 8, carbs 14, protein 11

86. Veggie Stew

Preparation time: 10 minutes

Cooking time: 20 minutes

Servings: 4

Ingredients:

1 tablespoon olive oil

1 cup fresh peas

1 yellow onion, chopped

1 zucchini, cubed

1 eggplant, cubed

1 green bell pepper, roughly cubed

1 red bell pepper, roughly cubed

1 cup cherry tomatoes, halved

2 cups corn

¼ cup celery, chopped

1 teaspoon thyme, chopped

2 teaspoons garlic, minced

Salt and black pepper to the taste

½ cup veggie stock

1 cup tomato sauce

1 tablespoon cilantro, chopped

Directions:

In your air fryer's pan, combine the peas with the onion, zucchini and the other ingredients, toss and cook at 380 degrees F for 20 minutes.

Divide into bowls and serve for lunch.

Nutrition: calories 286, fat 10, fiber 2, carbs 16, protein 11

87. Creamy Zucchini Mix

Preparation time: 10 minutes

Cooking time: 15 minutes

Servings: 4

Ingredients:

2 tablespoons olive oil

1 pound zucchinis, cut in medium wedges

1 yellow onion, chopped

1 cup heavy cream

Salt and black pepper to the taste

1 tablespoon balsamic vinegar

¼ teaspoon thyme, dried

Directions:

In your air fryer's pan, combine the zucchinis with the oil and the other ingredients, toss and cook at 360 degrees F for 15 minutes.

Divide between plates and serve for lunch.

Nutrition: calories 181, fat 4, fiber 4, carbs 10, protein 5

88. Pork and Tomatoes Mix

Preparation time: 10 minutes

Cooking time: 25 minutes

Servings: 4

Ingredients:

1 bunch kale, torn

1 pound pork stew meat, cubed

Salt and black pepper to the taste

1 cup tomatoes, cubed

1 tablespoon olive oil

1 teaspoon turmeric powder

1 teaspoon rosemary, dried

1 tablespoon chives, chopped

1 teaspoon sweet paprika

Directions:

Heat up the air fryer at 360 degrees F with the oil, add the meat and brown for 5 minutes.

Add the kale and the other ingredients, toss and cook for 20 minutes.

Divide the mix between plates and serve for lunch.

Nutrition: calories 210, fat 7, fiber 2, carbs 14, protein 5

89. Salsa Chicken

Preparation time: 10 minutes

Cooking time: 20 minutes

Servings: 4

Ingredients:

1 pound chicken breast, skinless, boneless and cubed

2 tablespoons olive oil

1 red onion, chopped

½ cup cilantro, chopped

½ cup green onions, chopped

2 cups salsa

2 teaspoons chili powder

1 teaspoon cumin, ground

Directions:

Heat up the air fryer with the oil at 370 degrees F, add the onion and the meat and cook for 5 minutes.

Add the other ingredients, toss and cook for 15 minutes more.

Divide the mix between plates and serve for lunch

Nutrition: calories 285, fat 12, fiber 6, carbs 22, protein 15

90. Eggplant and Tomato Stew

Preparation time: 5 minutes

Cooking time: 15 minutes

Servings: 4

Ingredients:

2 tablespoons olive oil

1 red onion, chopped

1 pound eggplant, cubed

½ pound cherry tomatoes, halved

1 cup tomato sauce

1 tablespoon basil, chopped

1 tablespoon chives, chopped

1 teaspoon chili powder

1 teaspoon cumin, ground

Salt and black pepper to the taste

Directions:

In your air fryer's pan, combine the eggplant with the onion, tomatoes and the other ingredients, toss and cook at 360 degrees F for 15 minutes.

Divide the stew into bowls and serve.

Nutrition: calories 200, fat 9, fiber 2, carbs 9, protein 12

91. Roasted Cauliflower Cream

Preparation time: 10 minutes

Cooking time: 20 minutes

Servings: 4

Ingredients:

1 pound cauliflower florets

1 tablespoon olive oil

1 teaspoon turmeric powder

2 cups hot veggie stock

1 cup heavy cream

1 teaspoon garlic powder

1 teaspoon rosemary, dried

Salt and black pepper to the taste

Directions:

In your air fryer's basket, combine the cauliflower with the oil, turmeric, garlic powder and rosemary, toss and cook at 360 degrees F for 20 minutes.

Transfer the cauliflower to a blender, add the remaining ingredients, pulse well, divide into bowls and serve for lunch.

Nutrition: calories 270, fat 8, fiber 12, carbs 17, protein 12

92. Garlic Pork Bowls

Preparation time: 10 minutes

Cooking time: 25 minutes

Servings: 4

Ingredients:

1 pound pork tenderloin, cubed

3 garlic cloves, minced

¼ cup balsamic vinegar

1 tablespoon olive oil

1 cup baby kale

1 cup tomatoes, cubed

A pinch of salt and black pepper

1 teaspoon cumin, ground

½ teaspoon fennel seeds, crushed

Directions:

Heat up the air fryer with the oil at 370 degrees F, add the garlic, onion and the meat and cook for 5 minutes.

Add the rest of the ingredients, toss and cook for 20 minutes more.

Divide the mix into bowls and serve for lunch.

Nutrition: calories 290, fat 7, fiber 9, carbs 17, protein 9

93. Peas Stew

Preparation time: 10 minutes

Cooking time: 20 minutes

Servings: 4

Ingredients:

2 cups fresh peas

1 tomato, cubed

1 red onion, sliced

1 red bell pepper, chopped

1 cup tomato sauce

1 cup veggie stock

Salt and black pepper to the taste

1 tablespoon olive oil

1 tablespoon dill, chopped

Directions:

1. In your air fryer's pan, combine the peas with the onion, tomato and the other ingredients, toss and cook at 400 degrees F for 20 minutes, stirring halfway.

2. Divide into bowls and serve for lunch.

Nutrition: calories 280, fat 12, fiber 2, carbs 16, protein 11

94. Beef and Sauce

Preparation time: 5 minutes

Cooking time: 25 minutes

Servings: 4

Ingredients:

2 pounds beef stew meat, cubed

1 yellow onion, chopped

2 tablespoons BBQ sauce

1 teaspoon chili powder

1 teaspoon smoked paprika

A pinch of salt and black pepper

1 cup tomato passata

1 teaspoon rosemary, dried

1 teaspoon coriander, ground

A pinch of salt and black pepper

Directions:

In your air fryer's pan, combine the beef with the onion, bbq sauce and the other ingredients, toss and cook at 380 degrees F for 25 minutes.

Divide the mix into bowls and serve.

Nutrition: calories 251, fat 14, fiber 8, carbs 16, protein 8

95. Ginger Lamb Mix

Preparation time: 10 minutes

Cooking time: 30 minutes

Servings: 4

Ingredients:

1 tablespoon olive oil

1 tablespoon ginger, grated

1 pound lamb shoulder, cubed

1 yellow onion, chopped

1 tablespoon rosemary, chopped

1 cup tomato passata

2 tablespoons walnuts, chopped

1 and ½ pounds rack of lamb

Salt and black pepper to the taste

Directions:

In your air fryer's pan, combine the lamb with the ginger, oil and the other ingredients, toss and cook at 380 degrees F for 30 minutes.

Serve for lunch right away.

Nutrition: calories 251, fat 8, fiber 6, carbs 16, protein 9

96. Cod and Broccoli Mix

Preparation time: 5 minutes

Cooking time: 15 minutes

Servings: 4

Ingredients:

1 pound cod fillets, boneless and roughly cubed

1 cup broccoli florets

4 scallions, chopped

1 tablespoon balsamic vinegar

Juice of ½ lemon

1 tablespoon olive oil

Salt and black pepper to the taste

3 garlic cloves, minced

½ tablespoon cilantro, chopped

Directions:

Heat up the air fryer with the oil at 350 degrees F, add the scallions and the cod and cook for 5 minutes.

Add the other ingredients, toss gently and cook for 10 minutes.

Divide everything between plates and serve.

Nutrition: calories 251, fat 7, fiber 4, carbs 9, protein 5

97. Chicken and Corn Stew

Preparation time: 6 minutes

Cooking time: 20 minutes

Servings: 4

Ingredients:

1 pound chicken breast, skinless, boneless and cubed

1 cup fresh corn

1 yellow onion, chopped

1 red bell pepper, chopped

2 garlic cloves, minced

1 cup canned tomatoes, roughly cubed

1 cup veggie stock

Salt and black pepper to the taste

½ teaspoons chili powder

1 tablespoon cilantro, chopped

Directions:

In your air fryer's pan, combine the chicken with the corn and the other ingredients, toss and cook at 370 degrees F for 20 minutes.

Divide into bowls and serve for lunch.

Nutrition: calories 251, fat 9, fiber 5, carbs 14, protein 4

98. Oregano Turkey Bowls

Preparation time: 10 minutes

Cooking time: 25 minutes

Servings: 4

Ingredients:

1 pound turkey breast, skinless, boneless and cubed

2 yellow onions, sliced

1 cup tomatoes, cubed

1 cup canned artichoke hearts, drained and quartered

1 tablespoon balsamic vinegar

1 cup tomato sauce

1 cup baby spinach

1 tablespoon garlic, minced

1 tablespoon balsamic vinegar

Salt and black pepper to the taste

2 tablespoons oregano, chopped

Directions:

In your air fryer's pan, combine the turkey with the onions, tomatoes and the other ingredients, toss and cook at 380 degrees F for 25 minutes shaking the machine from time to time.

Divide the mix into bowls and serve for lunch.

Nutrition: calories 200, fat 4, fiber 5, carbs 16, protein 6

99. Rice and Beans Mix

Preparation time: 5 minutes

Cooking time: 25 minutes

Servings: 4

Ingredients:

1 cup wild rice

1 cup canned red kidney beans, drained and rinsed

2 cups veggie stock

1 tablespoon olive oil

1 yellow onion, chopped

1 red chili, chopped

1 tomato, cubed

2 garlic cloves, minced

1 teaspoon ginger, grated

½ teaspoon oregano, dried

Salt and black pepper to the taste

1 tablespoon chives, chopped

Directions:

In a pan that fits your air fryer, combine the rice with the stock, the beans and the other ingredients, toss and cook at 360 degrees F for 25 minutes.

Divide the mix into bowls and serve for lunch.

Nutrition: calories 200, fat 8, fiber 4, carbs 8, protein 3

100. Green Beans Stew

Preparation time: 10 minutes

Cooking time: 20 minutes

Servings: 4

Ingredients:

1 pound green beans, trimmed and halved

1 red onion, chopped

1 tablespoon olive oil

1 tablespoon balsamic vinegar

1 cup canned tomatoes, chopped

½ cup tomato sauce

1 green bell pepper, chopped

1 tablespoon chili powder

¼ teaspoon sweet paprika

Salt and black pepper to the taste

2 tablespoons dill, chopped

Directions:

In a pan that fits your air fryer, combine the green beans with the onion, oil and the other ingredients, toss and cook at 380 degrees F for 20 minutes.

Divide the stew into bowls and serve for lunch right away.

Nutrition: calories 200, fat 8, fiber 4, carbs 9, protein 4

101. Turkey and Fennel Stew

Preparation time: 10 minutes

Cooking time: 25 minutes

Servings: 4

Ingredients:

1 pound turkey breast, skinless, boneless and cubed

1 fennel bulb, sliced

2 carrots, sliced

1 yellow onion, chopped

2 tablespoons olive oil

1 cup tomato sauce

1 teaspoon chili powder

1 tablespoon thyme, chopped

Salt and black pepper to the taste

1 tablespoon cilantro, chopped

Directions:

In your air fryer's pan, combine the meat with the fennel and the other ingredients, toss and cook at 365 degrees F for 25 minutes.

Divide the stew into bowls and serve.

Nutrition: calories 200, fat 8, fiber 2, carbs 8, protein 6

102. Spinach and Chickpeas Stew

Preparation time: 5 minutes

Cooking time: 20 minutes

Servings: 4

Ingredients:

2 cups canned chickpeas, drained and rinsed

1 cup baby spinach

1 red onion, chopped

2 garlic cloves, minced

1 tablespoon avocado oil

Salt and black pepper to the taste

1 cup veggie stock

1 cup tomato sauce

1 tablespoon sweet paprika

Directions:

In your air fryer's pan, combine the chickpeas with the spinach and the other ingredients, toss and cook at 370 degrees F for 20 minutes.

Divide the stew into bowls and serve for lunch.

Nutrition: calories 200, fat 8, fiber 3, carbs 15, protein 5

103. Potato Curry

Preparation time: 5 minutes

Cooking time: 25 minutes

Servings: 4

Ingredients:

4 gold potatoes, peeled and roughly cubed

1 yellow onion, chopped

1 tablespoon olive oil

1 tablespoon garlic, minced

10 ounces baby spinach

1 cup tomatoes, cubed

1 teaspoon ginger, grated

1 tablespoon lemon juice

2 tablespoons yellow curry paste

2 tablespoons cilantro, chopped

Salt and black pepper to the taste

Directions:

In your air fryer's pan, combine the potatoes with the onion, oil and the other ingredients, toss and cook at 370 degrees F for 25 minutes.

Divide into bowls and serve for lunch.

Nutrition: calories 251, fat 6, fiber 8, carbs 16, protein 7

104. Lamb and Eggplant Stew

Preparation time: 5 minutes

Cooking time: 30 minutes

Servings: 4

Ingredients:

1 red onion, chopped

1 pound lamb shoulder, cubed

2 eggplants, cubed

1 cup canned tomatoes, chopped

2 teaspoons rosemary, dried

1 teaspoon coriander powder

Salt and black pepper to the taste

2 red bell peppers, cubed

1 tablespoon parsley, chopped

Juice of ½ lime

Zest of 1 lime, grated

Directions:

In your air fryer's pan, combine the lamb with the onion, eggplants and the other ingredients, toss and cook at 370 degrees F for 30 minutes.

Divide into bowls and serve for lunch.

Nutrition: calories 251, fat 7, fiber 6, carbs 14, protein 9

105. Salmon and Okra Mix

Preparation time: 5 minutes

Cooking time: 15 minutes

Servings: 4

Ingredients:

4 salmon fillets, boneless

1 cup okra, sliced

1 cup tomatoes, cubed

1 red onion, chopped

2 tablespoons olive oil

2 garlic cloves, minced

1 teaspoon turmeric powder

1 teaspoon thyme, dried

Salt and black pepper to the taste

1 tablespoon chives, chopped

Directions:

In your air fryer's pan, combine the salmon with the okra, tomatoes and the other ingredients, toss gently and cook at 370 degrees F for 15 minutes.

Divide the mix between plates and serve for lunch.

Nutrition: calories 181, fat 7, fiber 4, carbs 9, protein 6

106. Beef and Green Beans

Preparation time: 5 minutes

Cooking time: 30 minutes

Servings: 4

Ingredients:

1 tablespoon olive oil

1 pound beef stew meat, cubed

2 cups green beans, trimmed and halved

1 green chili, chopped

1 yellow onion, chopped

1 teaspoon chili powder

1 cup tomato sauce

½ teaspoon turmeric powder

Salt and black pepper to the taste

3 garlic cloves, minced

1 tablespoon cilantro, chopped

Directions:

In your air fryer's pan, combine the meat with the oil, green beans and the other ingredients, toss and cook at 370 degrees F for 30 minutes.

Divide the mix into bowls and serve for lunch.

Nutrition: calories 251, fat 7, fiber 7, carbs 14, protein 6

107. Chicken Thighs and Onions Mix

Preparation time: 10 minutes

Cooking time: 25 minutes

Servings: 4

Ingredients:

2 pounds chicken thighs, skinless and boneless

2 red onions, chopped

4 scallions, chopped

Salt and black pepper to the taste

1 teaspoon garlic powder

1 cup chicken stock

1 cup canned tomatoes, chopped

1 tablespoon cilantro, chopped

1 teaspoon sweet paprika

Directions:

In your air fryer, combine the chicken thighs with the onions, scallions and the other ingredients, toss and cook at 380 degrees F for 25 minutes shaking the machine halfway.

Divide the mix between plates and serve for lunch.

Nutrition: calories 261, fat 7, fiber 4, carbs 9, protein 15

108. Basil Cod Mix

Preparation time: 10 minutes

Cooking time: 15 minutes

Servings: 4

Ingredients:

2 pounds cod fillets, boneless

2 scallions, chopped

1 tablespoon avocado oil

Juice of 1 lime

Salt and black pepper to the taste

2 tablespoons tomato paste

½ cup basil, chopped

2 teaspoons sweet paprika

Directions:

In your air fryer, combine the cod with the oil, scallions and the other ingredients, toss gently and cook at 380 degrees F for 15 minutes.

Divide between plates and serve for lunch.

Nutrition: calories 200, fat 7, fiber 6, carbs 16, protein 14

109. Baby Carrots Stew

Preparation time: 10 minutes

Cooking time: 20 minutes

Servings: 4

Ingredients:

1 pound baby carrots

1 yellow onion, chopped

2 tablespoons avocado oil

1 cup tomato paste

1 teaspoon chili powder

Salt and black pepper to the taste

2 tablespoons butter, melted

1 cup chicken stock

2 tablespoon dill, chopped

Directions:

In your air fryer, combine the carrots with the onion and the other ingredients, toss and cook 380 degrees F for 20 minutes.

Divide into bowls and serve for lunch.

Nutrition: calories 100, fat 3, fiber 3, carbs 8, protein 8

110. Shrimp and Chickpeas Mix

Preparation time: 10 minutes

Cooking time: 12 minutes

Servings: 4

Ingredients:

1 cup canned chickpeas, drained and rinsed

1 pound shrimp, peeled and deveined

1 tablespoon avocado oil

1 cup baby spinach

1 cup tomatoes, cubed

1 teaspoon rosemary, dried

1 teaspoon cumin, ground

Salt and black pepper to the taste

Directions:

In your air fryer, combine the chickpeas with the shrimp and the other ingredients, toss and cook at 380 degrees F for 12 minutes.

Divide into bowls and serve for lunch.

Nutrition: calories 200, fat 6, fiber 9, carbs 11, protein 6

Chapter 4.Seafood recipes

111.Salmon and Green Olives

Preparation Time: 20 minutes
Servings: 4

Ingredients:

4 salmon fillets; boneless

1 cup green olives, pitted and sliced

1/3 cup olive oil

1 tbsp. lemon zest; grated

Juice of 2 limes

Salt and black pepper to taste.

Directions:

In a baking dish that fits your air fryer, mix all the ingredients, toss, put the pan in the fryer and cook at 370°F for 15 minutes.

Divide everything between plates and serve.

Nutrition: Calories: 204; Fat: 12g; Fiber: 3g; Carbs: 5g; Protein: 15g

112. Cod Fillets

Preparation Time: 20 minutes
Servings: 4

Ingredients:

4 cod fillets; boneless

1 fennel; sliced

2 garlic cloves; minced

1 red bell pepper; chopped.

2 tbsp. olive oil

1 tbsp. thyme; chopped.

½ tsp. black peppercorns

2 tsp. Italian seasoning

A pinch of salt and black pepper

Directions:

Take a bowl and mix the fennel with bell pepper and the other ingredients except the fish fillets and toss.

Put this into a pan that fits the air fryer, add the fish on top

Introduce the pan in your air fryer and cook at 380°F for 15 minutes. Divide between plates and serve.

Nutrition: Calories: 241; Fat: 12g; Fiber: 4g; Carbs: 7g; Protein: 11g

113. Fish and Salsa

Preparation Time: 20 minutes
Servings: 4

Ingredients:

4 sea bass fillets; boneless

3 garlic cloves; minced

3 tomatoes; roughly chopped.

2 spring onions; chopped.

¼ cup chicken stock

1 tbsp. balsamic vinegar

1 tbsp. olive oil

A pinch of salt and black pepper

Directions:

In a blender, combine all the ingredients except the fish and pulse well.

Put the mix in a pan that fits the air fryer, add the fish, toss gently, introduce the pan in the fryer and cook at 380°F for 15 minutes. Divide between plates and serve.

Nutrition: Calories: 261; Fat: 11g; Fiber: 4g; Carbs: 7g; Protein: 11g

114. Trout Fillets and Bell Peppers

Preparation Time: 21 minutes
Servings: 2

Ingredients:

2 trout fillets; boneless

1 red bell pepper; chopped.

2 garlic cloves; minced

2 tomatoes; cubed

2 tbsp. almond flakes

1 tbsp. balsamic vinegar

1 tbsp. olive oil

A pinch of salt and black pepper

Directions:

Arrange the fish in a pan that fits your air fryer, add the rest of the ingredients and toss gently.

Cook at 370°F for 16 minutes, divide between plates and serve

Nutrition: Calories: 261; Fat: 14g; Fiber: 5g; Carbs: 6g; Protein: 14g

115. Sea Bass and Risotto

Preparation Time: 20 minutes
Servings: 4

Ingredients:

4 sea bass fillets; boneless

1 cup cauliflower rice

½ cup chicken stock

1 garlic clove; minced

1 tbsp. parmesan; grated

1 tbsp. chervil; chopped.

1 tbsp. parsley; chopped.

1 tbsp. tarragon; chopped.

1 tbsp. ghee; melted

A pinch of salt and black pepper

Directions:

In a pan that fits your air fryer, mix the cauliflower rice with the stock, parmesan, chervil, tarragon and parsley, toss, introduce the pan in the air fryer and cook at 380°F for 12 minutes

Take a bowl and mix the fish with salt, pepper, garlic and melted ghee and toss gently

Put the fish over the cauliflower rice, cook at 380°F for 12 minutes more, divide everything between plates and serve.

Nutrition: Calories: 261; Fat: 12g; Fiber: 4g; Carbs: 6g; Protein: 11g

116. Shrimp Kebabs

Preparation Time: 17 minutes
Servings: 2

Ingredients:

½ medium red bell pepper; cut into 1-inch-thick squares

18 medium shelled and deveined shrimp

¼ medium red onion; cut into 1-inch-thick squares

1 medium zucchini; cut into 1-inch cubes

1½ tbsp. coconut oil; melted

2 tsp. chili powder

½ tsp. paprika

¼ tsp. ground black pepper

Directions:

Soak four 6-inch bamboo skewers in water for 30 minutes. Place a shrimp on the skewer, then a zucchini, a pepper and an onion. Repeat until all ingredients are utilized

Brush each kebab with coconut oil. Sprinkle with chili powder, paprika and black pepper. Place kebabs into the air fryer basket

Adjust the temperature to 400 Degrees F and set the timer for 7 minutes or until shrimp is fully cooked and veggies are tender. Flip kebabs halfway through the cooking time. Serve warm.

Nutrition: Calories: 166; Protein: 9.5g; Fiber: 3.1g; Fat: 10.7g; Carbs: 8.5g

117. Simple Shrimp

Preparation Time: 13 minutes
Servings: 4

Ingredients:

1 lb. shrimp; peeled and deveined

1 cup chicken stock

1 tbsp. red onion; chopped.

2 tbsp. olive oil

Directions:

In a pan that fits your air fryer, mix the shrimp with the oil, onion and the stock.

Introduce the pan in the fryer and cook at 380°F for 10 minutes. Divide into bowls and serve

Nutrition: Calories: 261; Fat: 6g; Fiber: 8g; Carbs: 16g; Protein: 6g

118. Spicy Avocado Cod

Preparation Time: 20 minutes
Servings: 2

Ingredients:

1 medium avocado; peeled, pitted and sliced

¼ cup chopped pickled jalapeños.

2 (3-oz.cod fillets

½ medium lime

1 cup shredded cabbage

¼ cup full-fat sour cream.

2 tbsp. full-fat mayonnaise

½ tsp. paprika

¼ tsp. garlic powder.

1 tsp. chili powder

1 tsp. cumin

Directions:

Take a large bowl, place cabbage, sour cream, mayonnaise and jalapeños. Mix until fully coated. Let sit for 20 minutes in the refrigerator

Sprinkle cod fillets with chili powder, cumin, paprika and garlic powder. Place each fillet into the air fryer basket. Adjust the temperature to 370 Degrees F and set the timer for 10 minutes.

Flip the fillets halfway through the cooking time. When fully cooked, fish should have an internal temperature of at least 145 Degrees F

To serve, divide slaw mixture into two serving bowls, break cod fillets into pieces and spread over the bowls and top with avocado. Squeeze lime juice over each bowl. Serve immediately.

Nutrition: Calories: 342; Protein: 16.1g; Fiber: 6.4g; Fat: 25.2g; Carbs: 11.7g

119. Shrimp Scampi

Preparation Time: 18 minutes
Servings: 4

Ingredients:

1 lb. medium peeled and deveined shrimp

½ medium lemon.

¼ cup heavy whipping cream.

1 tbsp. chopped fresh parsley

4 tbsp. salted butter

¼ tsp. xanthan gum

¼ tsp. red pepper flakes

1 tsp. minced roasted garlic

Directions:

In a medium saucepan over medium heat, melt butter. Zest the lemon, then squeeze juice into the pan. Add garlic

Pour in the cream, xanthan gum and red pepper flakes. Whisk until the mixture begins to thicken, about 2–3 minutes

Place shrimp into a 4-cup round baking dish. Pour the cream sauce over the shrimp and cover with foil. Place the dish into the air fryer basket.

Adjust the temperature to 400 Degrees F and set the timer for 8 minutes. Stir twice during cooking. When done, garnish with parsley and serve warm.

Nutrition: Calories: 240; Protein: 16.7g; Fiber: 0.4g; Fat: 17.0g; Carbs: 2.4g

120. Paprika Cod

Preparation Time: 19 minutes
Servings: 4

Ingredients:

4 cod fillets; boneless

1 tbsp. olive oil

2 tsp. sweet paprika

Juice of 1 lime

Salt and black pepper to taste.

Directions:

Take a bowl and mix all the ingredients, transfer the fish to your air fryer's basket and cook 350°F for 7 minutes on each side

Divide the fish between plates and serve with a side salad.

Nutrition: Calories: 240; Fat: 14g; Fiber: 2g; Carbs: 4g; Protein: 16g

121. Roasted Char Fillets

Preparation Time: 23 minutes
Servings: 4

Ingredients:

4 char fillets; boneless

1 fennel bulb; sliced with a mandoline

½ cup dill; chopped.

5 garlic cloves; minced

2 tbsp. balsamic vinegar

1 tbsp. lemon juice

1 tbsp. lemon peel; grated

3 tbsp. olive oil

1 tsp. caraway seeds

A pinch of salt and black pepper

Directions:

In a pan that fits your air fryer, mix the fish with all the other ingredients, toss, introduce in the air fryer and cook at 390°F for 18 minutes.

Divide the fish between plates and serve with a side salad.

Nutrition: Calories: 251; Fat: 16g; Fiber: 4g; Carbs: 6g; Protein: 13g

122. Buttery Shrimp

Preparation Time: 11 minutes
Servings: 2

Ingredients:

8 oz. medium shelled and deveined shrimp

2 tbsp. salted butter; melted.

¼ tsp. onion powder.

½ tsp. garlic powder.

½ tsp. Old Bay seasoning

1 tsp. paprika

Directions:

Toss all ingredients together in a large bowl. Place shrimp into the air fryer basket.

Adjust the temperature to 400 Degrees F and set the timer for 6 minutes. Turn the shrimp halfway through the cooking time to ensure even cooking. Serve immediately.

Nutrition: Calories: 192; Protein: 16.6g; Fiber: 0.5g; Fat: 11.9g; Carbs: 2.5g

123. Crab Legs

Preparation Time: 20 minutes
Servings: 4

Ingredients:

3 lb. crab legs

¼ cup salted butter; melted and divided

Juice of ½ medium lemon.

¼ tsp. garlic powder.

Directions:

Take a large bowl, drizzle 2 tbsp. butter over crab legs. Place crab legs into the air fryer basket.

Adjust the temperature to 400 Degrees F and set the timer for 15 minutes. Shake the air fryer basket to toss the crab legs halfway through the cooking time

In a small bowl, mix remaining butter, garlic powder and lemon juice

To serve, crack open crab legs and remove meat. Dip in lemon butter.

Nutrition: Calories: 123; Protein: 15.7g; Fiber: 0.0g; Fat: 5.6g; Carbs: 0.4g

124. Lime Trout and Shallots

Preparation Time: 17 minutes
Servings: 4

Ingredients:

4 trout fillets; boneless

3 garlic cloves; minced

6 shallots; chopped.

½ cup butter; melted

½ cup olive oil

Juice of 1 lime

A pinch of salt and black pepper

Directions:

In a pan that fits the air fryer, combine the fish with the shallots and the rest of the ingredients, toss gently

Put the pan in the machine and cook at 390°F for 12 minutes, flipping the fish halfway.

Divide between plates and serve with a side salad.

Nutrition: Calories: 270; Fat: 12g; Fiber: 4g; Carbs: 6g; Protein: 12g

125. Flounder Fillets and Mushrooms

Preparation Time: 20 minutes
Servings: 4

Ingredients:

4 flounder fillets; boneless

2 green onions; chopped.

2 cups mushrooms; sliced

2 tbsp. coconut aminos

2 tsp. olive oil

1 ½ tsp. ginger; grated

A pinch of salt and black pepper

Directions:

Heat u a pan that fits your air fryer with the oil over medium-high heat, add the mushrooms and all the other ingredients except the fish, toss and sauté for 5 minutes

Add the fish, toss gently, introduce the pan in the fryer and cook at 390°F for 10 minutes. Divide between plates and serve.

Nutrition: Calories: 271; Fat: 12g; Fiber: 4g; Carbs: 6g; Protein: 11g

126. Salmon Jerky

Preparation Time: 4 hours 5 minutes
Servings: 4

Ingredients:

1 lb. salmon, skin and bones removed

¼ cup soy sauce

½ tsp. ground ginger

¼ tsp. red pepper flakes

½ tsp. liquid smoke

¼ tsp. ground black pepper

Juice of ½ medium lime

Directions:

Slice salmon into ¼-inch-thick slices, 4-inch long

Place strips into a large storage bag or a covered bowl and add remaining ingredients. Allow to marinate for 2 hours in the refrigerator

Place each strip into the air fryer basket in a single layer. Adjust the temperature to 140 Degrees F and set the timer for 4 hours. Cool then store in a sealed container until ready to eat.

Nutrition: Calories: 108; Protein: 15.1g; Fiber: 0.2g; Fat: 4.1g; Carbs: 1.0g

127. Air Fried Tuna Salad Bites

Preparation Time: 17 minutes
Servings: 12 bites

Ingredients:

1 (10-oz.can tuna, drained

½ cup blanched finely ground almond flour, divided.

¼ cup full-fat mayonnaise

1 stalk celery; chopped

1 medium avocado; peeled, pitted and mashed

2 tsp. coconut oil

Directions:

Take a large bowl, mix tuna, mayonnaise, celery and mashed avocado. Form the mixture into balls.

Roll balls in almond flour and spritz with coconut oil. Place balls into the air fryer basket.

Adjust the temperature to 400 Degrees F and set the timer for 7 minutes.

Gently turn tuna bites after 5 minutes. Serve warm.

Nutrition: Calories: 323; Protein: 17.3g; Fiber: 4.0g; Fat: 25.4g; Carbs: 6.3g

128. Lemony Flounder Fillets

Preparation Time: 17 minutes
Servings: 2

Ingredients:

2 flounder fillets; boneless

2 garlic cloves; minced

2 tbsp. olive oil

2 tbsp. lemon juice

2 tsp. coconut aminos

½ tsp. stevia

A pinch of salt and black pepper

Directions:

In a pan that fits your air fryer, mix all the ingredients, toss, introduce in the fryer and cook at 390°F for 12 minutes. Divide into bowls and serve.

Nutrition: Calories: 251; Fat: 13g; Fiber: 3g; Carbs: 5g; Protein: 10g

129. Fish Fillets and Coconut Sauce

Preparation Time: 25 minutes
Servings: 4

Ingredients:

4 sea bass fillets; boneless

2 red chilies; minced

2 cups coconut cream

½ cup okra

2 tomatoes; cubed

2 spring onions; chopped.

Juice of 1 lime

1 garlic clove; minced

A handful coriander; chopped.

A pinch of salt and black pepper

Directions:

Put the coconut cream in a pan that fits the air fryer, add garlic, spring onions, lime juice, tomatoes, okra, chilies and the coriander, toss, bring to a simmer and cook for 5 - 6 minutes.

Add the fish, toss gently, introduce in the fryer and cook at 380°F for 15 minutes. Divide between plates and serve.

Nutrition: Calories: 261; Fat: 12g; Fiber: 5g; Carbs: 6g; Protein: 11g

130. Butter Trout

Preparation Time: 22 minutes
Servings: 4

Ingredients:

4 trout fillets; boneless

Juice of 1 lime

1 tbsp. parsley; chopped.

1 tbsp. chives; chopped.

4 tbsp. butter; melted

Salt and black pepper to taste.

Directions:

Mix the fish fillets with the melted butter, salt and pepper, rub gently, put the fish in your air fryer's basket and cook at 390°F for 6 minutes on each side.

Divide between plates and serve with lime juice drizzled on top and with parsley and chives sprinkled at the end.

Nutrition: Calories: 221; Fat: 11g; Fiber: 4g; Carbs: 6g; Protein: 9g

131. Black Sea Bass with Rosemary Vinaigrette

Preparation Time: 17 minutes
Servings: 4

Ingredients:

4 black sea bass fillets; boneless and skin scored

3 garlic cloves; minced

2 tbsp. olive oil

1 tbsp. rosemary; chopped.

3 tbsp. black olives, pitted and chopped.

A pinch of salt and black pepper

Juice of 1 lime

Directions:

Take a bowl and mix the oil with the olives and the rest of the ingredients except the fish and whisk well.

Place the fish in a pan that fits the air fryer, spread the rosemary vinaigrette all over.

Put the pan in the machine and cook at 380°F for 12 minutes, flipping the fish halfway. Divide between plates and serve

Nutrition: Calories: 220; Fat: 12g; Fiber: 4g; Carbs: 6g; Protein: 10g

132. Tuna Zoodle Casserole

Preparation Time: 30 minutes
Servings: 4

Ingredients:

1 oz. pork rinds, finely ground

2 medium zucchini, spiralized

2 (5-oz.cans albacore tuna

¼ cup diced white onion

¼ cup chopped white mushrooms

2 stalks celery, finely chopped

½ cup heavy cream

½ cup vegetable broth

2 tbsp. full-fat mayonnaise

2 tbsp. salted butter

½ tsp. red pepper flakes

¼ tsp. xanthan gum

Directions:

In a large saucepan over medium heat, melt butter. Add onion, mushrooms and celery and sauté until fragrant, about 3–5 minutes.

Pour in heavy cream, vegetable broth, mayonnaise and xanthan gum. Reduce heat and continue cooking an additional 3 minutes, until the mixture begins to thicken

Add red pepper flakes, zucchini and tuna. Turn off heat and stir until zucchini noodles are coated

Pour into 4-cup round baking dish. Top with ground pork rinds and cover the top of the dish with foil. Place into the air fryer basket. Adjust the temperature to 370 Degrees F and set the timer for 15 minutes.

When 3 minutes remain, remove the foil to brown the top of the casserole. Serve warm.

Nutrition: Calories: 339; Protein: 19.7g; Fiber: 1.8g; Fat: 25.1g; Carbs: 6.1g

133. Swordfish Steaks and Tomatoes

Preparation Time: 15 minutes
Servings: 2

Ingredients:

30 oz. canned tomatoes; chopped.

2 1-inch thick swordfish steaks

2 tbsp. capers, drained

1 tbsp. red vinegar

2 tbsp. oregano; chopped.

A pinch of salt and black pepper

Directions:

In a pan that fits the air fryer, combine all the ingredients, toss, put the pan in the fryer and cook at 390°F for 10 minutes, flipping the fish halfway

Divide the mix between plates and serve

Nutrition: Calories: 280; Fat: 12g; Fiber: 4g; Carbs: 6g; Protein: 11g

134. Crab Cakes

Preparation Time: 20 minutes
Servings: 4

Ingredients:

½ medium green bell pepper; seeded and chopped

¼ cup chopped green onion

1 large egg.

2 (6-oz.cans lump crabmeat

¼ cup blanched finely ground almond flour.

½ tbsp. lemon juice

2 tbsp. full-fat mayonnaise

½ tsp. Old Bay seasoning

½ tsp. Dijon mustard

Directions:

Take a large bowl, combine all ingredients. Form into four balls and flatten into patties. Place patties into the air fryer basket

Adjust the temperature to 350 Degrees F and set the timer for 10 minutes.

Flip patties halfway through the cooking time. Serve warm.

Nutrition: Calories: 151; Protein: 13.4g; Fiber: 0.9g; Fat: 10.0g; Carbs: 2.3g

135. Fish Sticks

Preparation Time: 25 minutes
Servings: 4

Ingredients:

1 lb. cod fillet; cut into 3/4-inch strips

1 oz. pork rinds, finely ground

1 large egg.

¼ cup blanched finely ground almond flour.

1 tbsp. coconut oil

½ tsp. Old Bay seasoning

Directions:

Place ground pork rinds, almond flour, Old Bay seasoning and coconut oil into a large bowl and mix together. Take a medium bowl, whisk egg

Dip each fish stick into the egg and then gently press into the flour mixture, coating as fully and evenly as possible. Place fish sticks into the air fryer basket

Adjust the temperature to 400 Degrees F and set the timer for 10 minutes or until golden. Serve immediately.

Nutrition: Calories: 205; Protein: 24.4g; Fiber: 0.8g; Fat: 10.7g; Carbs: 1.6g

136. Delicious Shrimp recipe

Preparation Time: 17 minutes
Servings: 4

Ingredients:

1 lb. medium shelled and deveined shrimp

¼ cup full-fat mayonnaise

2 tbsp. sriracha

2 tbsp. salted butter; melted.

¼ tsp. powdered erythritol

¼ tsp. garlic powder.

⅛ tsp. ground black pepper

½ tsp. Old Bay seasoning

Directions:

Take a large bowl, toss shrimp in butter, Old Bay seasoning and garlic powder. Place shrimp into the air fryer basket

Adjust the temperature to 400 Degrees F and set the timer for 7 minutes.

Flip the shrimp halfway through the cooking time. Shrimp will be bright pink when fully cooked

In another large bowl, mix sriracha, powdered erythritol, mayonnaise and pepper.

Toss shrimp in the spicy mixture and serve immediately.

Nutrition: Calories: 143; Protein: 16.4g; Fiber: 0.0g; Fat: 6.4g; Mg; Carbs: 3.0g

137. Salmon Patties

Preparation Time: 18 minutes
Servings: 2

Ingredients:

2 (5-oz.pouches cooked pink salmon

¼ cup ground pork rinds

1 large egg.

2 tbsp. full-fat mayonnaise

1 tsp. chili powder

2 tsp. sriracha

Directions:

Mix all ingredients in a large bowl and form into four patties. Place patties into the air fryer basket.

Adjust the temperature to 400 Degrees F and set the timer for 8 minutes. Carefully flip each patty halfway through the cooking time

Patties will be crispy on the outside when fully cooked.

Nutrition: Calories: 319; Protein: 33.8g; Fiber: 0.5g; Fat: 19.0g; Carbs: 1.9g

138. Trout and Almonds

Preparation Time: 20 minutes
Servings: 2

Ingredients:

2 trout fillets; boneless

1 tbsp. parsley; chopped.

1 tbsp. ghee; melted

1 tbsp. olive oil

2 tbsp. almonds, crushed

Zest of ½ lemon; grated

A pinch of salt and black pepper

Directions:

Take a bowl and mix the trout with all the other ingredients except the parsley and toss.

Put the fish in your air fryer's basket and cook at 370°F for 15 minutes, flipping the fillets halfway.

Divide between plates, sprinkle the parsley on top and serve.

Nutrition: Calories: 271; Fat: 13g; Fiber: 4g; Carbs: 6g; Protein: 12g

Chapter 5. Beef, pork and lamb recipes

139. Cumin Beef

Preparation time: 10 minutes

Cooking time: 25 minutes

Servings: 4

Ingredients:

2 pounds beef stew meat, cut into strips

2 tablespoons avocado oil

Juice of 1 lime

2 garlic cloves, minced

Salt and black pepper to the taste

2 tablespoons garlic powder

1 tablespoon cumin, ground

1 tablespoon chives, chopped

Directions:

Heat up the air fryer with the oil at 380 degrees F, add the meat, lime juice and the other ingredients, toss, cook for 25 minutes, divide between plates and serve with a side salad.

Nutrition: calories 453, fat 15.4, fiber 0.9, carbs 4.6, protein 70

140. Balsamic Beef and Broccoli

Preparation time: 10 minutes

Cooking time: 25 minutes

Servings: 4

Ingredients:

1 pound beef stew, cut into strips

1 cup broccoli florets

2 tablespoons balsamic vinegar

2 red onions, sliced

2 tablespoons olive oil

2 garlic cloves, minced

A pinch of salt and black pepper

Directions:

Heat up the air fryer with the oil at 390 degrees F, add the meat, onion, broccoli and the other ingredients, toss, cook for 25 minutes, divide into bowls and serve.

Nutrition: calories 201, fat 13.3, fiber 3.5, carbs 14.9, protein 7

141. Mustard Beef Mix

Preparation time: 10 minutes

Cooking time: 20 minutes

Servings: 4

Ingredients:

1 yellow onion, chopped

2 garlic cloves, minced

1 red bell pepper, cut into strips

2 pounds beef stew meat, cubed

1 green bell pepper, cut in strips

Salt and black pepper to the taste

1 teaspoon rosemary, dried

1 tablespoon mustard

1 tablespoon olive oil

1 cup beef stock

Directions:

In your air fryer's pan, combine the onion with the garlic, the meat and the other ingredients, toss well and cook at 400 degrees F for 20 minutes.

Divide the mix into bowls and serve.

Nutrition: calories 502, fat 18.8, fiber 2, carbs 8.8, protein 71.2

142. Garlic Pork Chops

Preparation time: 10 minutes

Cooking time: 20 minutes

Servings: 4

Ingredients:

1 pound pork chops

4 garlic cloves, minced

2 tablespoons avocado oil

Salt and black pepper to the taste

2 tablespoons dark soy sauce

A pinch of cayenne pepper

Directions:

In a bowl, combine the pork chops with the garlic and the other ingredients, toss, transfer them to the air fryer's basket and cook at 390 degrees F for 20 minutes flipping the chops halfway.

Divide everything between plates and serve.

Nutrition: calories 285, fat 8, fiber 2, carbs 18, protein 20

143. Mint Lamb Chops

Preparation time: 10 minutes

Cooking time: 20 minutes

Servings: 4

Ingredients:

2 tablespoons olive oil

1 pound lamb chops

2 tablespoons mint, chopped

Juice of 1 lime

Salt and black pepper to the taste

4 garlic cloves, minced

1 teaspoon sweet paprika

Directions:

In a bowl, mix the lamb chops with the oil, mint and the other ingredients, toss well, transfer them to the air fryer's basket and cook at 400 degrees F for 20 minutes.

Serve with a side salad.

Nutrition: calories 301, fat 7, fiber 5, carbs 19, protein 22

144. Beef and Walnuts Mix

Preparation time: 10 minutes

Cooking time: 20 minutes

Servings: 4

Ingredients:

2 tablespoons walnuts, chopped

2 tablespoons olive oil

2 pounds beef stew meat, cubed

2 garlic cloves, minced

2 tablespoons chives, chopped

Salt and black pepper to the taste

¼ cup beef stock

1 tablespoon oregano, chopped

Directions:

Heat up the air fryer with the oil at 380 degrees F, add the meat and garlic and cook for 5 minutes.

Add the rest of the ingredients, toss, cook for 15 minutes more, divide between plates and serve with a side salad.

Nutrition: calories 280, fat 12, fiber 8, carbs 20, protein 19

145. Creamy Pork Chops

Preparation time: 10 minutes

Cooking time: 25 minutes

Servings: 4

Ingredients:

2 pounds pork chops

2 tablespoons butter, melted

1 tablespoon coriander, chopped

2 cups heavy cream

2 garlic cloves, minced

1 shallot, chopped

Juice of ½ lime

Salt and black pepper to the taste

Directions:

In your air fryer's pan, combine the pork chops with the melted butter and the other ingredients, toss and cook at 380 degrees F for 25 minutes.

Divide everything between plates and serve.

Nutrition: calories 283, fat 11, fiber 9, carbs 22, protein 14

146. Lamb and Sprouts Mix

Preparation time: 10 minutes

Cooking time: 25 minutes

Servings: 4

Ingredients:

1 pound lamb stew meat, cubed

2 tablespoons olive oil

2 tablespoons chives, chopped

1 cup Brussels sprouts, trimmed and halved

4 scallions, chopped

Salt and black pepper to the taste

4 garlic cloves, minced

½ cup beef stock

Salt and black pepper to the taste

Directions:

In your air fryer's pan, combine the lamb with the oil and the other ingredients, toss, cook at 380 degrees F for 25 minutes, divide between plates and serve.

Nutrition: calories 280, fat 13, fiber 9, carbs 22, protein 18

147. Tarragon Pork

Preparation time: 10 minutes

Cooking time: 25 minutes

Servings: 4

Ingredients:

2 pounds pork stew meat, cubed

2 tablespoons avocado oil

1 tablespoon tarragon, chopped

Juice of 1 lime

2 garlic cloves, minced

2 tablespoons chives, chopped

2 tablespoons mustard

Salt and black pepper to the taste

Directions:

Heat up the air fryer with the oil at 380 degrees F, add the meat, tarragon and the other ingredients, toss and cook for 25 minutes.

Divide everything between plates and serve.

Nutrition: calories 280, fat 12, fiber 2, carbs 17, protein 14

148. Buttery Pork and Carrots

Preparation time: 10 minutes

Cooking time: 25 minutes

Servings: 4

Ingredients:

2 tablespoons butter, melted

3 garlic cloves, minced

2 pounds pork stew meat, cubed

2 carrots, peeled and sliced

Salt and black pepper to the taste

½ cup beef stock

2 tablespoons chives, chopped

Directions:

Heat up the air fryer with the butter at 380 degrees F, add the meat and the garlic and cook for 5 minutes.

Add the rest of the ingredients, toss, cook for 20 minutes more, divide between plates and serve.

Nutrition: calories 300, fat 11, fiber 4, carbs 18, protein 22

149. Pesto Lamb Chops

Preparation time: 10 minutes

Cooking time: 20 minutes

Servings: 4

Ingredients:

1 pound lamb chops

2 tablespoons avocado oil

2 tablespoons basil pesto

1 yellow onion, chopped

2 garlic cloves, minced

2 tablespoons sweet paprika

Salt and black pepper to the taste

2 tablespoons chives, chopped

Directions:

In a bowl, combine the lamb chops with the oil, pesto and the other ingredients, toss well, transfer to the air fryer's basket and cook for 20 minutes at 380 degrees F.

Divide everything between plates and serve hot.

Nutrition: calories 310, fat 8, fiber 10, carbs 19, protein 25

150. Roasted Rib Eye Steaks

Preparation Time: 29 minutes
Servings: 4

Ingredients:

4 rib eye steaks

1 tbsp. olive oil

1 tsp. rosemary; chopped

1 tsp. sweet paprika

1 tsp. cumin, ground

A pinch of salt and black pepper

Directions:

Take a bowl and mix the steaks with the rest of the ingredients, toss and put them in your air fryer's basket and cook at 380°F for 12 minutes on each side

Divide between plates and serve.

Nutrition: Calories: 283; Fat: 12g; Fiber: 3g; Carbs: 6g; Protein: 17g

151. Juicy Pork Chops

Preparation Time: 20 minutes
Servings: 2

Ingredients:

2 (4-oz.boneless pork chops

2 tbsp. unsalted butter, divided.

¼ tsp. ground black pepper

¼ tsp. dried oregano.

1 tsp. chili powder

½ tsp. cumin

½ tsp. garlic powder.

Directions:

In a small bowl, mix chili powder, garlic powder, cumin, pepper and oregano. Rub dry rub onto pork chops. Place pork chops into the air fryer basket. Adjust the temperature to 400 Degrees F and set the timer for 15 minutes

The internal temperature should be at least 145 Degrees F when fully cooked. Serve warm, each topped with 1 tbsp. butter.

Nutrition: Calories: 313; Protein: 24.4g; Fiber: 0.7g; Fat: 22.6g; Carbs: 1.8g

152. Lasagna Casserole

Preparation Time: 30 minutes
Servings: 4

Ingredients:

¾ cup low-carb no-sugar-added pasta sauce

1 lb. 80/20 ground beef; cooked and drained

½ cup full-fat ricotta cheese

¼ cup grated Parmesan cheese.

½ tsp. garlic powder.

1 tsp. dried parsley.

½ tsp. dried oregano.

1 cup shredded mozzarella cheese

Directions:

In a 4-cup round baking dish, pour ¼ cup pasta sauce on the bottom of the dish. Place ¼ of the ground beef on top of the sauce.

In a small bowl, mix ricotta, Parmesan, garlic powder, parsley and oregano. Place dollops of half the mixture on top of the beef

Sprinkle with ⅓ of the mozzarella. Repeat layers until all beef, ricotta mixture, sauce and mozzarella are used, ending with the mozzarella on top

Cover dish with foil and place into the air fryer basket. Adjust the temperature to 370 Degrees F and set the timer for 15 minutes. In the last 2 minutes of cooking, remove the foil to brown the cheese. Serve immediately.

Nutrition: Calories: 371; Protein: 31.4g; Fiber: 1.6g; Fat: 21.4g; Carbs: 5.8g

153. Pulled Pork

Preparation Time: 2 hours
Servings: 8

Ingredients:

1 (4-poundpork shoulder

2 tbsp. chili powder

½ tsp. ground black pepper

½ tsp. cumin

½ tsp. onion powder.

1 tsp. garlic powder.

Directions:

In a small bowl, mix chili powder, garlic powder, onion powder, pepper and cumin. Rub the spice mixture over the pork shoulder, patting it into the skin

Place pork shoulder into the air fryer basket. Adjust the temperature to 350 Degrees F and set the timer for 150 minutes.

Pork skin will be crispy and meat easily shredded with two forks when done. The internal temperature should be at least 145 Degrees F

Nutrition: Calories: 537; Protein: 42.6g; Fiber: 0.8g; Fat: 35.5g; Carbs: 1.5g

154. Seasoned Lamb

Preparation Time: 40 minutes
Servings: 4

Ingredients:

1 lb. lamb leg; boneless and sliced

½ cup walnuts; chopped

2 garlic cloves; minced

1 tbsp. parsley; chopped

1 tbsp. rosemary; chopped

2 tbsp. olive oil

¼ tsp. red pepper flakes

½ tsp. mustard seeds

½ tsp. Italian seasoning

A pinch of salt and black pepper

Directions:

Take a bowl and mix the lamb with all the ingredients except the walnuts and parsley, rub well, put the slices your air fryer's basket and cook at 370°F for 35 minutes, flipping the meat halfway

Divide between plates, sprinkle the parsley and walnuts on top and serve with a side salad

Nutrition: Calories: 283; Fat: 13g; Fiber: 4g; Carbs: 6g; Protein: 15g

155. Pork Roast

Preparation Time: 35 minutes
Servings: 4

Ingredients:

1 lb. pork tenderloin, trimmed

2 tbsp. balsamic vinegar

3 tbsp. mustard

2 tbsp. olive oil

A pinch of salt and black pepper

Directions:

Take a bowl and mix the pork tenderloin with the rest of the ingredients and rub well.

Put the roast in your air fryer's basket and cook at 380°F for 30 minutes. Slice the roast, divide between plates and serve.

Nutrition: Calories: 274; Fat: 13g; Fiber: 4g; Carbs: 7g; Protein: 22

156. BBQ Meatballs

Preparation Time: 24 minutes
Servings: 4

Ingredients:

¼ lb. ground Italian sausage

1 lb. 80/20 ground beef.

4 slices sugar-free bacon; cooked and chopped

¼ cup chopped white onion

¼ cup chopped pickled jalapeños.

½ cup low-carb, sugar-free barbecue sauce

1 large egg.

1 tsp. dried parsley.

¼ tsp. onion powder.

½ tsp. garlic powder.

Directions:

Take a large bowl, mix ground beef, sausage and egg until fully combined. Mix in all remaining ingredients except barbecue sauce. Form into eight meatballs. Place meatballs into the air fryer basket.

Adjust the temperature to 400 Degrees F and set the timer for 14 minutes

Turn the meatballs halfway through the cooking time

When done, meatballs should be browned on the outside and have an internal temperature of at least 180 Degrees F. Remove meatballs from fryer and toss in barbecue sauce. Serve warm.

Nutrition: Calories: 336; Protein: 28.1g; Fiber: 0.4g; Fat: 19.5g; Carbs: 4.4g

157. Lamb Cakes

Preparation Time: 35 minutes
Servings: 8

Ingredients:

2 ½ lb. lamb meat, ground

2 spring onions; chopped

½ cup almond meal

3 eggs, whisked

1 tbsp. garlic; minced

2 tbsp. cilantro; chopped

Zest of 1 lemon

Juice of 1 lemon

Cooking spray

2 tbsp. mint; chopped

A pinch of salt and black pepper

Directions:

Take a bowl and mix all the ingredients except the cooking spray, stir well and shape medium cakes out of this mix

Put the cakes in your air fryer, grease them with cooking spray and cook at 390°F for 15 minutes on each side

Divide between plates and serve with a side salad

Nutrition: Calories: 283; Fat: 13g; Fiber: 4g; Carbs: 6g; Protein: 15g

158. Lamb Chops and Mint Sauce

Preparation Time: 29 minutes
Servings: 4

Ingredients:

8 lamb chops

1 cup mint; chopped

1 garlic clove; minced

2 tbsp. olive oil

Juice of 1 lemon

A pinch of salt and black pepper

Directions:

In a blender, combine all the ingredients except the lamb and pulse well.

Rub lamb chops with the mint sauce, put them in your air fryer's basket and cook at 400°F for 12 minutes on each side

Divide everything between plates and serve.

Nutrition: Calories: 284; Fat: 14g; Fiber: 3g; Carbs: 6g; Protein: 16g

159. Easy Pork Chops

Preparation Time: 25 minutes
Servings: 4

Ingredients:

1½ oz. pork rinds, finely ground

1 tsp. chili powder

½ tsp. garlic powder.

1 tbsp. coconut oil; melted

4 (4-oz.pork chops

Directions:

Take a large bowl, mix ground pork rinds, chili powder and garlic powder.

Brush each pork chop with coconut oil and then press into the pork rind mixture, coating both sides. Place each coated pork chop into the air fryer basket

Adjust the temperature to 400 Degrees F and set the timer for 15 minutes. Flip each pork chop halfway through the cooking time

When fully cooked the pork chops will be golden on the outside and have an internal temperature of at least 145 Degrees F.

Nutrition: Calories: 292; Protein: 29.5g; Fiber: 0.3g; Fat: 18.5g; Carbs: 0.6g

160. Roasted Spare Ribs

Preparation Time: 50 minutes
Servings: 4

Ingredients:

2 racks of ribs

1 tbsp. coriander; chopped

2 tbsp. cocoa powder

½ tsp. chili powder

½ tsp. cumin, ground

½ tsp. cinnamon powder

Cooking spray

A pinch of salt and black pepper

Directions:

Grease the ribs with the cooking spray, mix with the other ingredients and rub very well.

Put the ribs in your air fryer's basket and cook at 390°F for 45 minutes. Divide between plates and serve with a side salad

Nutrition: Calories: 284; Fat: 14g; Fiber: 5g; Carbs: 7g; Protein: 20g

161. Beef Tenderloin

Preparation Time: 35 minutes
Servings: 6

Ingredients:

1 (2-poundbeef tenderloin, trimmed of visible fat

2 tbsp. salted butter; melted.

2 tsp. minced roasted garlic

3 tbsp. ground 4-peppercorn blend

Directions:

In a small bowl, mix the butter and roasted garlic. Brush it over the beef tenderloin.

Place the ground peppercorns onto a plate and roll the tenderloin through them, creating a crust. Place tenderloin into the air fryer basket

Adjust the temperature to 400 Degrees F and set the timer for 25 minutes. Turn the tenderloin halfway through the cooking time. Allow meat to rest 10 minutes before slicing.

Nutrition: Calories: 289; Protein: 34.7g; Fiber: 0.9g; Fat: 13.8g; Carbs: 2.5g

162. Lamb Skewers

Preparation Time: 30 minutes
Servings: 4

Ingredients:

2 lb. lamb meat; cubed

2 red bell peppers; cut into medium pieces

¼ cup olive oil

2 tbsp. lemon juice

1 tbsp. oregano; dried

1 tbsp. red vinegar

1 tbsp. garlic; minced

½ tsp. rosemary; dried

A pinch of salt and black pepper

Directions:

Take a bowl and mix all the ingredients and toss them well.

Thread the lamb and bell peppers on skewers, place them in your air fryer's basket and cook at 380°F for 10 minutes on each side. Divide between plates and serve with a side salad

Nutrition: Calories: 274; Fat: 12g; Fiber: 3g; Carbs: 6g; Protein: 16g

163. Basil Pork Chops

Preparation Time: 30 minutes
Servings: 4

Ingredients:

4 pork chops

2 tsp. basil; dried

½ tsp. chili powder

2 tbsp. olive oil

A pinch of salt and black pepper

Directions:

In a pan that fits your air fryer, mix all the ingredients, toss.

Introduce in the fryer and cook at 400°F for 25 minutes. Divide everything between plates and serve

Nutrition: Calories: 274; Fat: 13g; Fiber: 4g; Carbs: 6g; Protein: 18g

164. Beef and Radishes

Preparation Time: 20 minutes
Servings: 2

Ingredients:

1 lb. radishes, quartered

2 cups corned beef, cooked and shredded

2 spring onions; chopped

2 garlic cloves; minced

A pinch of salt and black pepper

Directions:

In a pan that fits your air fryer, mix the beef with the rest of the ingredients, toss.

Put the pan in the fryer and cook at 390°F for 15 minutes

Divide everything into bowls and serve.

Nutrition: Calories: 267; Fat: 13g; Fiber: 2g; Carbs: 5g; Protein: 15g

165. Fajita Flank Steak Rolls

Preparation Time: 35 minutes
Servings: 6

Ingredients:

2 lb. flank steak

4 (1-oz.slices pepper jack cheese

1 medium red bell pepper; seeded and sliced into strips

¼ cup diced yellow onion

1 medium green bell pepper; seeded and sliced into strips

2 tbsp. unsalted butter.

1 tsp. cumin

½ tsp. garlic powder.

2 tsp. chili powder

Directions:

In a medium skillet over medium heat, melt butter and begin sautéing onion, red bell pepper and green bell pepper. Sprinkle with chili powder, cumin and garlic powder. Sauté until peppers are tender, about 5–7 minutes.

Lay flank steak flat on a work surface. Spread onion and pepper mixture over entire steak rectangle. Lay slices of cheese on top of onions and peppers, barely overlapping

With the shortest end toward you, begin rolling the steak, tucking the cheese down into the roll as necessary.

Secure the roll with twelve toothpicks, six on each side of the steak roll. Place steak roll into the air fryer basket

Adjust the temperature to 400 Degrees F and set the timer for 15 minutes. Rotate the roll halfway through the cooking time. Add an additional 1–4 minutes depending on your preferred internal temperature (135 Degrees F for medium

When timer beeps, allow roll to rest 15 minutes, then slice into six even pieces. Serve warm.

Nutrition: Calories: 439; Protein: 38.0g; Fiber: 1.2g; Fat: 26.6g; Carbs: 3.7g

166. Crusted Lamb Cutlets

 Preparation Time: 35 minutes
Servings: 4

Ingredients:

8 lamb cutlets

¼ cup parmesan, grated

½ cup coconut flakes

2 tbsp. parsley; chopped

2 tbsp. chives; chopped

3 tbsp. olive oil

1 tbsp. rosemary; chopped

3 tbsp. mustard

A pinch of salt and black pepper

Directions:

Take a bowl and mix the lamb cutlets with all the ingredients except the parmesan and the coconut flakes and toss well.

Dredge the cutlets in parmesan and coconut flakes, put them in your air fryer's basket and cook at 390°F for 15 minutes on each side

Divide between plates and serve.

Nutrition: Calories: 284; Fat: 13g; Fiber: 3g; Carbs: 6g; Protein: 17g

167. Rosemary Roasted Lamb Cutlets

Preparation Time: 35 minutes
Servings: 4

Ingredients:

8 lamb cutlets

2 garlic cloves; minced

2 tbsp. rosemary; chopped

2 tbsp. olive oil

A pinch of salt and black pepper

A pinch of cayenne pepper

Directions:

Take a bowl and mix the lamb with the rest of the ingredients and rub well.

Put the lamb in the fryer's basket and cook at 380°F for 30 minutes, flipping them halfway. Divide the cutlets between plates and serve

Nutrition: Calories: 274; Fat: 12g; Fiber: 3g; Carbs: 5g; Protein: 15g

168. Spicy Beef

Preparation Time: 25 minutes
Servings: 4

Ingredients:

4 beef steaks

1 tbsp. hot paprika

1 tbsp. butter; melted

Salt and black pepper to taste.

Directions:

Take a bowl and mix the beef with the rest of the ingredients, rub well, transfer the steaks to your air fryer's basket and cook at 390°F for 10 minutes on each side

Divide the steaks between plates and serve with a side salad.

Nutrition: Calories: 280; Fat: 12g; Fiber: 4g; Carbs: 6g; Protein: 17g

169. Herbed Lamb

Preparation Time: 40 minutes
Servings: 4

Ingredients:

8 lamb cutlets

¼ cup mustard

2 garlic cloves; minced

1 tbsp. oregano; chopped

1 tbsp. mint chopped.

1 tbsp. chives; chopped

1 tbsp. basil; chopped

A drizzle of olive oil

A pinch of salt and black pepper

Directions:

Take a bowl and mix the lamb with the rest of the ingredients and rub well.

Put the cutlets in your air fryer's basket and cook at 380°F for 15 minutes on each side

Divide between plates and serve with a side salad.

Nutrition: Calories: 284; Fat: 13g; Fiber: 3g; Carbs: 6g; Protein: 14g

170. Smoked Lamb Chops

Preparation Time: 25 minutes
Servings: 4

Ingredients:

4 lamb chops

4 garlic cloves; minced

2 tbsp. olive oil

¼ tsp. smoked paprika

½ tsp. chili powder

A pinch of salt and black pepper

Directions:

Take a bowl and mix the lamb with the rest of the ingredients and toss well

Transfer the chops to your air fryer's basket and cook at 390°F for 10 minutes on each side. Serve with a side salad

Nutrition: Calories: 274; Fat: 12g; Fiber: 4g; Carbs: 6g; Protein: 17g

171. Moroccan Lamb

Preparation Time: 35 minutes
Servings: 4

Ingredients:

8 lamb cutlets

½ cup mint leaves

6 garlic cloves

3 tbsp. lemon juice

1 tbsp. coriander seeds

4 tbsp. olive oil

1 tbsp. cumin, ground

Zest of 2 lemons, grated

A pinch of salt and black pepper

Directions:

In a blender, combine all the ingredients except the lamb and pulse well.

Rub the lamb cutlets with this mix, place them in your air fryer's basket and cook at 380°F for 15 minutes on each side. Serve with a side salad

Nutrition: Calories: 284; Fat: 13g; Fiber: 3g; Carbs: 5g; Protein: 15g

172. Greek Lamb Chops

Preparation Time: 35 minutes
Servings: 4

Ingredients:

4 lamb chops

1 cup Greek yogurt

2 tbsp. coconut oil; melted

½ tsp. turmeric powder

1 tsp. lemon zest, grated

A pinch of salt and black pepper

Directions:

Take a bowl and mix the lamb chops with the rest of the ingredients and toss well.

Put the chops in your air fryer's basket and cook at 380°F for 15 minutes on each side

Divide between plates and serve

Nutrition: Calories: 283; Fat: 13g; Fiber: 3g; Carbs: 6g; Protein: 15g

173. Beef and Chorizo Burger

Preparation Time: 25 minutes
Servings: 4

Ingredients:

5 slices pickled jalapeños; chopped

¼ lb. Mexican-style ground chorizo

¾lb. 80/20 ground beef.

¼ cup chopped onion

¼ tsp. cumin

1 tsp. minced garlic

2 tsp. chili powder

Directions:

Take a large bowl, mix all ingredients. Divide the mixture into four sections and form them into burger patties.

Place burger patties into the air fryer basket, working in batches if necessary. Adjust the temperature to 375 Degrees F and set the timer for 15 minutes

Flip the patties halfway through the cooking time. Serve warm.

Nutrition: Calories: 291; Protein: 21.6g; Fiber: 0.9g; Fat: 18.3g; Carbs: 4.7g

174. Lamb and Pine Nuts Meatballs

Preparation Time: 35 minutes
Servings: 4

Ingredients:

1 ½ lb. lamb, ground

2 garlic cloves; minced

1 egg, whisked

1 scallion; chopped

½ cup pine nuts, toasted and chopped.

1 tbsp. olive oil

1 tbsp. thyme; chopped

A pinch of salt and black pepper

Directions:

Take a bowl and mix the lamb with the rest of the ingredients except the oil, stir well and shape medium meatballs out of this mix

Grease the meatballs with the oil, put them in your air fryer's basket and cook at 380°F for 15 minutes on each side. Divide between plates and serve with a side salad

Nutrition: Calories: 287; Fat: 12g; Fiber: 3g; Carbs: 6g; Protein: 17g

175. Lamb Loin and Tomato Vinaigrette

Preparation Time: 40 minutes
Servings: 4

Ingredients:

4 lamb loin slices

3 garlic cloves; minced

1/3 cup parsley; chopped

1/3 cup sun-dried tomatoes; chopped

2 tbsp. balsamic vinegar

2 tbsp. water

2 tbsp. olive oil

2 tsp. thyme; chopped

A pinch of salt and black pepper

Directions:

In a blender, combine all the ingredients except the lamb slices and pulse well.

Take a bowl and mix the lamb with the tomato vinaigrette and toss well

Put the lamb in your air fryer's basket and cook at 380°F for 15 minutes on each side

Divide everything between plates and serve.

Nutrition: Calories: 273; Fat: 13g; Fiber: 4g; Carbs: 6g; Protein: 17g

176. Beef and Broccoli Stir-Fry

Preparation Time: 1 hour 20 minutes
Servings: 2

Ingredients:

½ lb. sirloin steak, thinly sliced

2 tbsp. soy sauce (or liquid aminos

¼ tsp. grated ginger

¼ tsp. finely minced garlic

1 tbsp. coconut oil

2 cups broccoli florets

¼ tsp. crushed red pepper

⅛ tsp. xanthan gum

½ tsp. sesame seeds

Directions:

To marinate beef, place it into a large bowl or storage bag and add soy sauce, ginger, garlic and coconut oil. Allow to marinate for 1 hour in refrigerator.

Remove beef from marinade, reserving marinade and place beef into the air fryer basket. Adjust the temperature to 320 Degrees F and set the timer for 20 minutes

After 10 minutes, add broccoli and sprinkle red pepper into the fryer basket and shake.

Pour the marinade into a skillet over medium heat and bring to a boil, then reduce to simmer. Stir in xanthan gum and allow to thicken

When air fryer timer beeps, quickly empty fryer basket into skillet and toss. Sprinkle with sesame seeds. Serve immediately.

Nutrition: Calories: 342; Protein: 27.0g; Fiber: 2.7g; Fat: 18.9g; Carbs: 9.6g

177. Pork Chop Salad

Preparation Time: 23 minutes
Servings: 2

Ingredients:

2 (4-oz.pork chops; chopped into 1-inch cubes

½ cup shredded Monterey jack cheese

1 medium avocado; peeled, pitted and diced

¼ cup full-fat ranch dressing

4 cups chopped romaine

1 medium Roma tomato; diced

1 tbsp. chopped cilantro

1 tbsp. coconut oil

½ tsp. garlic powder.

¼ tsp. onion powder.

2 tsp. chili powder

1 tsp. paprika

Directions:

Take a large bowl, drizzle coconut oil over pork. Sprinkle with chili powder, paprika, garlic powder and onion powder. Place pork into the air fryer basket.

Adjust the temperature to 400 Degrees F and set the timer for 8 minutes. Pork will be golden and crispy when fully cooked

Take a large bowl, place romaine, tomato and crispy pork. Top with shredded cheese and avocado. Pour ranch dressing around bowl and toss the salad to evenly coat. Top with cilantro. Serve immediately.

Nutrition: Calories: 526; Protein: 34.4g; Fiber: 8.6g; Fat: 37.0g; Carbs: 13.8g

178. Crispy Chicken Tenders

Preparation Time: 25 minutes
Servings: 4

Ingredients:

9 oz. coconut flakes

4 chicken breasts, skinless; boneless and cut into tenders

1/3 cup almond flour

2 eggs, whisked

A pinch of salt and black pepper

Directions:

Season the chicken tenders with salt and pepper, dredge them in almond flour, then dip in eggs and roll in coconut flakes.

Put the chicken tenders in your air fryer's basket and cook at 400°F for 10 minutes on each side.

Divide between plates and serve with a side salad.

Nutrition: Calories: 250; Fat: 12g; Fiber: 4g; Carbs: 6g; Protein: 15g

179. Spinach Stuffed Chicken Breast

Preparation Time: 40 minutes
Servings: 2

Ingredients:

5 oz. frozen spinach, thawed and drained

¼ cup chopped yellow onion

¼ cup crumbled feta

2 (6-oz.boneless, skinless chicken breasts

1 tbsp. coconut oil

1 tbsp. unsalted butter.

½ tsp. garlic powder, divided.

½ tsp. salt, divided.

Directions:

In a medium skillet over medium heat, add butter to the pan and sauté spinach 3 minutes. Sprinkle ¼ tsp. garlic powder. and ¼ tsp. salt onto spinach and add onion to the pan.

Continue sautéing 3 more minutes, then remove from heat and place in medium bowl. Fold feta into spinach mixture.

Slice a roughly 4-inch slit into the side of each chicken breast, lengthwise. Spoon half of the mixture into each piece and secure closed with a couple toothpicks

Sprinkle outside of chicken with remaining garlic powder and salt. Drizzle with coconut oil. Place chicken breasts into the air fryer basket.

Adjust the temperature to 350 Degrees F and set the timer for 25 minutes

When completely cooked chicken should be golden brown and have an internal temperature of at least 165 Degrees F. Slice and serve warm.

Nutrition: Calories: 393; Protein: 43.9g; Fiber: 2.5g; Fat: 18.5g; Carbs: 6.2g

180. Mozzarella Chicken Breasts

Preparation Time: 29 minutes
Servings: 6

Ingredients:

1 lb. mozzarella; sliced

2 tomatoes; sliced

2 cups baby spinach

6 chicken breasts, skinless; boneless and halved

2 tbsp. olive oil

1 tbsp. basil; chopped

1 tsp. Italian seasoning

A pinch of salt and black pepper

Directions:

Make slits in each chicken breast halves, season with salt, pepper and Italian seasoning and stuff with mozzarella, spinach and tomatoes.

Drizzle the oil over stuffed chicken, put it in your air fryer's basket and cook at 370°F for 12 minutes on each side. Divide between plates and serve with basil sprinkled on top.

Nutrition: Calories: 285; Fat: 12g; Fiber: 4g; Carbs: 7g; Protein: 15g

181. Chicken Wings and Pesto

Preparation Time: 35 minutes
Servings: 4

Ingredients:

1 ½ lb. chicken wings

1 cup basil pesto

2 tbsp. olive oil

A pinch of salt and black pepper

Directions:

Take a bowl and mix the chicken wings with all the ingredients and toss well.

Put the meat in the air fryer's basket and cook at 380°F for 25 minutes

Divide between plates and serve.

Nutrition: Calories: 244; Fat: 11g; Fiber: 4g; Carbs: 6g; Protein: 17g

182. Cardamom Duck Legs

Preparation Time: 35 minutes
Servings: 4

Ingredients:

4 duck legs

Zest of ½ lemon, grated

Juice of ½ lemon

2 tbsp. almonds, toasted and chopped.

2 tbsp. olive oil

1 tbsp. cardamom, crushed

¼ tsp. allspice

Directions:

Take a bowl and mix the duck legs with the remaining ingredients except the almonds and toss.

Put the duck legs in your air fryer's basket and cook at 380°F for 15 minutes on each side

Divide the duck legs between plates, sprinkle the almonds on top and serve with a side salad.

Nutrition: Calories: 284; Fat: 12g; Fiber: 4g; Carbs: 6g; Protein: 18g

183. Spiced Chicken Breasts

Preparation Time: 25 minutes
Servings: 4

Ingredients:

4 chicken breasts, skinless and boneless

1 tbsp. parsley; chopped

1 tsp. smoked paprika

1 tsp. garlic powder

1 tsp. chili powder

A drizzle of olive oil

A pinch of salt and black pepper

Directions:

Season chicken with salt and pepper and rub it with the oil and all the other ingredients except the parsley

Put the chicken breasts in your air fryer's basket and cook at 350°F for 10 minutes on each side

Divide between plates, sprinkle the parsley on top and serve

Nutrition: Calories: 222; Fat: 11g; Fiber: 4g; Carbs: 6g; Protein: 12g

184. Spiced Duck Legs

Preparation Time: 30 minutes
Servings: 4

Ingredients:

4 duck legs

2 garlic cloves; minced

2 tbsp. olive oil

1 tsp. five spice

1 tsp. hot chili powder

A pinch of salt and black pepper

Directions:

Take a bowl and mix the duck legs with all the other ingredients and rub them well.

Put the duck legs in your air fryer's basket and cook at 380°F for 25 minutes, flipping them halfway

Divide between plates and serve

Nutrition: Calories: 287; Fat: 12g; Fiber: 4g; Carbs: 6g; Protein: 17g

185. Mustard Turkey Bites

Preparation Time: 25 minutes
Servings: 4

Ingredients:

1 big turkey breast, skinless; boneless and cubed

4 garlic cloves; minced

1 tbsp. mustard

1 ½ tbsp. olive oil

Salt and black pepper to taste.

Directions:

Take a bowl and mix the chicken with the garlic and the other ingredients and toss.

Put the turkey in your air fryer's basket, cook at 360°F for 20 minutes, divide between plates and serve with a side salad

Nutrition: Calories: 240; Fat: 12g; Fiber: 4g; Carbs: 6g; Protein: 15g

186. Nutmeg Chicken Thighs

Preparation Time: 35 minutes
Servings: 4

Ingredients:

2 lb. chicken thighs

2 tbsp. olive oil

½ tsp. nutmeg, ground

A pinch of salt and black pepper

Directions:

Season the chicken thighs with salt and pepper and rub with the rest of the ingredients

Put the chicken thighs in air fryer's basket, cook at 360°F for 15 minutes on each side, divide between plates and serve.

Nutrition: Calories: 271; Fat: 12g; Fiber: 4g; Carbs: 6g; Protein: 13g

187. Creamy Chicken Wings

Preparation Time: 35 minutes
Servings: 4

Ingredients:

2 lb. chicken wings

¼ cup parmesan, grated

½ cup heavy cream

3 garlic cloves; minced

3 tbsp. butter; melted

½ tsp. oregano; dried

½ tsp. basil; dried

Salt and black pepper to taste.

Directions:

In a baking dish that fits your air fryer, mix the chicken wings with all the ingredients except the parmesan and toss

Put the dish to your air fryer and cook at 380°F for 30 minutes. Sprinkle the cheese on top, leave the mix aside for 10 minutes, divide between plates and serve

Nutrition: Calories: 270; Fat: 12g; Fiber: 3g; Carbs: 6g; Protein: 17g

188. Chicken Stir-Fry

Preparation Time: 30 minutes
Servings: 2

Ingredients:

1 (6-oz.chicken breast; cut into 1-inch cubes

½ medium red bell pepper; seeded and chopped

½ medium zucchini; chopped

¼ medium red onion; peeled.and sliced

1 tbsp. coconut oil

½ tsp. garlic powder.

1 tsp. dried oregano.

¼ tsp. dried thyme

Directions:

Place all ingredients into a large mixing bowl and toss until the coconut oil coats the meat and vegetables. Pour the contents of the bowl into the air fryer basket

Adjust the temperature to 375 Degrees F and set the timer for 15 minutes. Shake the fryer basket halfway through the cooking time to redistribute the food. Serve immediately.

Nutrition: Calories: 186; Protein: 20.4g; Fiber: 1.7g; Fat: 8.0g; Carbs: 5.6g

189. Cheddar Turkey Bites

Preparation Time: 25 minutes
Servings: 4

Ingredients:

1 big turkey breast, skinless; boneless and cubed

1 tbsp. olive oil

¼ cup cheddar cheese, grated

¼ tsp. garlic powder

Salt and black pepper to taste.

Directions:

Rub the turkey cubes with the oil, season with salt, pepper and garlic powder and dredge in cheddar cheese.

Put the turkey bits in your air fryer's basket and cook at 380°F for 20 minutes. Divide between plates and serve with a side salad

Nutrition: Calories: 240; Fat: 11g; Fiber: 2g; Carbs: 5g; Protein: 12g

190. Chicken Parmesan

Preparation Time: 35 minutes
Servings: 4

Ingredients:

2 (6-oz.boneless, skinless chicken breasts

1 oz. pork rinds, crushed

½ cup grated Parmesan cheese, divided.

1 cup low-carb, no-sugar-added pasta sauce.

1 cup shredded mozzarella cheese, divided.

4 tbsp. full-fat mayonnaise, divided.

½ tsp. garlic powder.

¼ tsp. dried oregano.

½ tsp. dried parsley.

Directions:

Slice each chicken breast in half lengthwise and lb. out to 3/4-inch thickness. Sprinkle with garlic powder, oregano and parsley

Spread 1 tbsp. mayonnaise on top of each piece of chicken, then sprinkle ¼ cup mozzarella on each piece.

In a small bowl, mix the crushed pork rinds and Parmesan. Sprinkle the mixture on top of mozzarella

Pour sauce into 6-inch round baking pan and place chicken on top. Place pan into the air fryer basket. Adjust the temperature to 320 Degrees F and set the timer for 25 minutes

Cheese will be browned and internal temperature of the chicken will be at least 165 Degrees F when fully cooked. Serve warm.

Nutrition: Calories: 393; Protein: 34.2g; Fiber: 2.1g; Fat: 22.8g; Carbs: 6.8g

191. Lemon Pepper Drumsticks

Preparation Time: 30 minutes
Servings: 8 drumsticks

Ingredients:

8 chicken drumsticks

1 tbsp. lemon pepper seasoning

4 tbsp. salted butter; melted.

2 tsp. baking powder.

½ tsp. garlic powder.

Directions:

Sprinkle baking powder and garlic powder over drumsticks and rub into chicken skin. Place drumsticks into the air fryer basket.

Adjust the temperature to 375 Degrees F and set the timer for 25 minutes

Use tongs to turn drumsticks halfway through the cooking time. When skin is golden and internal temperature is at least 165 Degrees F, remove from fryer

Take a large bowl, mix butter and lemon pepper seasoning. Add drumsticks to the bowl and toss until coated. Serve warm.

Nutrition: Calories: 532; Protein: 48.3g; Fiber: 0.0g; Fat: 32.3g; Carbs: 1.2g

192. Chicken Pizza Crust

Preparation Time: 35 minutes
Servings: 4

Ingredients:

1 lb. ground chicken thigh meat

½ cup shredded mozzarella

¼ cup grated Parmesan cheese.

Directions:

Take a large bowl, mix all ingredients. Separate into four even parts.

Cut out four (6-inchcircles of parchment and press each portion of the chicken mixture out onto one of the circles. Place into the air fryer basket, working in batches as needed

Adjust the temperature to 375 Degrees F and set the timer for 25 minutes. Flip the crust halfway through the cooking time

Once fully cooked, you may top it with cheese and your favorite toppings and cook 5 additional minutes. Or, you may place crust into refrigerator or freezer and top when ready to eat.

Nutrition: Calories: 230; Protein: 24.7g; Fiber: 0.0g; Fat: 12.8g; Carbs: 1.2g

193. Spinach, Chicken and Feta Bites

Preparation Time: 22 minutes
Servings: 4

Ingredients:

1 lb. ground chicken thigh meat

½ oz. pork rinds, finely ground

⅓ cup crumbled feta

⅓ cup frozen spinach, thawed and drained

½ tsp. garlic powder.

¼ tsp. onion powder.

Directions:

Mix all ingredients in a large bowl. Roll into 2-inch balls and place into the air fryer basket, working in batches if needed

Adjust the temperature to 350 Degrees F and set the timer for 12 minutes. When done, internal temperature will be 165 Degrees F. Serve immediately.

Nutrition: Calories: 220; Protein: 24.1g; Fiber: 0.4g; Fat: 12.2g; Carbs: 1.5g

194. Turkey and Almonds

Preparation Time: 30 minutes
Servings: 2

Ingredients:

1 big turkey breast, skinless; boneless and halved

2 shallots; chopped

1/3 cup almonds; chopped

1 tbsp. sweet paprika

2 tbsp. olive oil

Salt and black pepper to taste.

Directions:

In a pan that fits the air fryer, combine the turkey with all the other ingredients, toss.

Put the pan in the machine and cook at 370°F for 25 minutes

Divide everything between plates and serve.

Nutrition: Calories: 274; Fat: 12g; Fiber: 3g; Carbs: 5g; Protein: 14g

195. Turkey and Spinach

Preparation Time: 20 minutes
Servings: 4

Ingredients:

1 lb. turkey meat, ground and browned

4 cups spinach leaves

1 tbsp. ginger, grated

2 tbsp. coconut aminos

1 tbsp. garlic; minced

A pinch of salt and black pepper

Directions:

In a pan that fits your air fryer, combine all the ingredients and toss.

Put the pan in the air fryer and cook at 380°F for 15 minutes Divide everything into bowls and serve

Nutrition: Calories: 240; Fat: 12g; Fiber: 3g; Carbs: 5g; Protein: 13g

196. Teriyaki Wings

Preparation Time: 1 hour 25 minutes
Servings: 4

Ingredients:

2 lb. chicken wings

½ cup sugar-free teriyaki sauce

2 tsp. baking powder.

¼ tsp. ground ginger

2 tsp. minced garlic

Directions:

Place all ingredients except baking powder into a large bowl or bag and let marinade for 1 hour in the refrigerator

Place wings into the air fryer basket and sprinkle with baking powder. Gently rub into wings.

Adjust the temperature to 400 Degrees F and set the timer for 25 minutes. Toss the basket two or three times during cooking

Wings should be crispy and cooked to at least 165 Degrees F internally when done. Serve immediately.

Nutrition: Calories: 446; Protein: 41.8g; Fiber: 0.1g; Fat: 29.8g; Carbs: 3.2g

197. Turkey Breasts and Celery

Preparation Time: 35 minutes
Servings: 4

Ingredients:

1 big turkey breast, skinless; boneless and sliced

4 garlic cloves; minced

4 celery stalks, roughly chopped.

3 tbsp. olive oil

1 tbsp. smoked paprika

1 tbsp. garlic powder

1 tsp. cumin, ground

1 tsp. turmeric powder

Directions:

In a pan that fits the air fryer, combine the turkey and the other ingredients, toss.

Put the pan in the machine and cook at 380°F for 30 minutes

Divide everything between plates and serve.

Nutrition: Calories: 285; Fat: 12g; Fiber: 3g; Carbs: 6g; Protein: 16g

198. Turkey and Rosemary Butter

Preparation Time: 29 minutes
Servings: 4

Ingredients:

1 turkey breast, skinless; boneless and cut into 4 pieces

2 tbsp. rosemary; chopped

2 tbsp. butter; melted

Juice of 1 lemon

A pinch of salt and black pepper

Directions:

Take a bowl and mix the butter with the rosemary, lemon juice, salt and pepper and whisk really well.

Brush the turkey pieces with the rosemary butter, put them your air fryer's basket, cook at 380°F for 12 minutes on each side. Divide between plates and serve with a side salad

Nutrition: Calories: 236; Fat: 12g; Fiber: 4g; Carbs: 6g; Protein: 13g

199. Cumin Turkey

Preparation Time: 30 minutes
Servings: 4

Ingredients:

1 lb. turkey meat; cubed and browned

12 oz. veggies stock

1 cup tomatoes; chopped

1 green bell pepper; chopped

3 garlic cloves; chopped

1 ½ tsp. cumin, ground

A pinch of salt and black pepper

Directions:

In a pan that fits your air fryer, mix the turkey with the rest of the ingredients, toss.

Put the pan in the machine and cook at 380°F for 25 minutes. Divide into bowls and serve

Nutrition: Calories: 274; Fat: 12g; Fiber: 4g; Carbs: 6g; Protein: 15g

200. Marinated Drumsticks

Preparation Time: 40 minutes
Servings: 4

Ingredients:

2 lb. chicken drumsticks

1 ½ cups tomato sauce

1 tbsp. coconut aminos

1 tsp. onion powder

½ tsp. chili powder

A pinch of salt and black pepper

Directions:

In bowl, mix the chicken drumsticks with all the other ingredients, toss and keep in the fridge for 10 minutes.

Drain the drumsticks, put them in your air fryer's basket and cook at 380°F for 15 minutes on each side. Divide everything between plates and serve

Nutrition: Calories: 254; Fat: 14g; Fiber: 4g; Carbs: 6g; Protein: 15g

201. Italian Chicken Thighs

Preparation Time: 25 minutes
Servings: 2

Ingredients:

4 bone-in, skin-on chicken thighs

2 tbsp. unsalted butter; melted.

¼ tsp. onion powder.

¼ tsp. dried oregano.

1 tsp. dried parsley.

½ tsp. garlic powder.

1 tsp. dried basil

Directions:

Brush chicken thighs with butter and sprinkle remaining ingredients over thighs. Place thighs into the air fryer basket.

Adjust the temperature to 380 Degrees F and set the timer for 20 minutes. Halfway through the cooking time, flip the thighs

When fully cooked, internal temperature will be at least 165 Degrees F and skin will be crispy.

Nutrition: Calories: 596; Protein: 68.3g; Fiber: 0.4g; Fat: 30.9g; Carbs: 1.2g

202. Asian Fried Chicken

Preparation Time: 40 minutes
Servings: 4

Ingredients:

2 (6-oz.boneless, skinless chicken breasts

2 oz. pork rinds, finely ground

1 tbsp. chili powder

2 tbsp. hot sauce

¼ tsp. onion powder.

¼ tsp. ground black pepper

½ tsp. cumin

Directions:

Slice each chicken breast in half lengthwise. Place the chicken into a large bowl and coat with hot sauce.

In a small bowl, mix chili powder, cumin, onion powder and pepper. Sprinkle over chicken

Place the ground pork rinds into a large bowl and dip each piece of chicken into the bowl, coating as much as possible. Place chicken into the air fryer basket

Adjust the temperature to 350 Degrees F and set the timer for 25 minutes. Halfway through the cooking time, carefully flip the chicken.

When done, internal temperature will be at least 165 Degrees F and pork rind coating will be dark golden brown.

Nutrition: Calories: 192; Protein: 27.8g; Fiber: 0.9g; Fat: 6.9g; Carbs: 1.6g

203. Smoked Chicken Wings

Preparation Time: 35 minutes
Servings: 4

Ingredients:

2 lb. chicken wings

1 tbsp. olive oil

1 tbsp. lime juice

1 tsp. red pepper flakes, crushed

2 tsp. smoked paprika

Salt and black pepper to taste.

Directions:

Take a bowl and mix the chicken wings with all the other ingredients and toss well

Put the chicken wings in your air fryer's basket and cook at 380°F for 15 minutes on each side. Divide between plates and serve with a side salad.

Nutrition: Calories: 280; Fat: 13g; Fiber: 3g; Carbs: 6g; Protein: 14g

204. Thyme Roasted Chicken

Preparation Time: 70 minutes
Servings: 6

Ingredients:

1 medium lemon.

1 (4-poundchicken

2 tbsp. salted butter; melted.

½ tsp. onion powder.

2 tsp. dried parsley.

1 tsp. baking powder.

2 tsp. dried thyme

1 tsp. garlic powder.

Directions:

Rub chicken with thyme, garlic powder, onion powder, parsley and baking powder.

Slice lemon and place four slices on top of chicken, breast side up and secure with toothpicks. Place remaining slices inside of the chicken

Place entire chicken into the air fryer basket, breast side down. Adjust the temperature to 350 Degrees F and set the timer for 60 minutes. After 30 minutes, flip chicken so breast side is up

When done, internal temperature should be 165 Degrees F and the skin golden and crispy. To serve, pour melted butter over entire chicken.

Nutrition: Calories: 504; Protein: 32.0g; Fiber: 0.3g; Fat: 36.8g; Carbs: 1.4g

205. Chicken Cheese Sticks

Preparation Time: 13 minutes
Servings: 2

Ingredients:

1 cup shredded cooked chicken

1 large egg.

¼ cup crumbled feta

1 cup shredded mozzarella cheese

¼ cup buffalo sauce

Directions:

Take a large bowl, mix all ingredients except the feta. Cut a piece of parchment to fit your air fryer basket and press the mixture into a ½-inch-thick circle

Sprinkle the mixture with feta and place into the air fryer basket. Adjust the temperature to 400 Degrees F and set the timer for 8 minutes

After 5 minutes, flip over the cheese mixture. Allow to cool 5 minutes before cutting into sticks. Serve warm.

Nutrition: Calories: 369; Protein: 35.7g; Fiber: 0.0g; Fat: 21.5g; Carbs: 2.2g

206. Jalapeño Chicken Thighs

Preparation Time: 25 minutes
Servings: 4

Ingredients

4 chicken thighs, boneless

2 garlic cloves, crushed

1 jalapeno pepper, finely chopped

4 tbsp chili sauce

Salt and black pepper

Directions

In a bowl, add thighs, garlic, jalapeno, chili sauce, salt, and black pepper, and stir to coat. Arrange the thighs in an even layer inside your air fryer and cook for 12 minutes at 360 F, turning once halfway through.

207. Easy Chicken Fingers with Parmesan

Preparation Time: 1 hour 30 minutes
Servings: 2

Ingredients

2 skinless and boneless chicken breasts, cut strips

1 tbsp salt

1 tbsp black pepper

2 cloves garlic, crushed

3 tbsp cornstarch

4 tbsp breadcrumbs, like flour bread

4 tbsp grated Parmesan cheese

2 eggs, beaten

Directions

Mix salt, garlic, and pepper in a bowl. Add the chicken and stir to coat. Marinate for an hour in the fridge.

Meanwhile, mix the breadcrumbs with cheese evenly; set aside. Remove the chicken from the fridge, lightly toss in cornstarch, dip in egg and coat them gently in the cheese mixture. Preheat the Air Fryer to 350 F.

Lightly spray the air fryer basket with cooking spray and place the chicken inside; cook for 15 minutes, until nice and crispy. Serve the chicken with a side of vegetable fries and cheese dip.

208. Chicken with Soy Sauce

Preparation Time: 1 hour 35 minutes
Servings: 3

Ingredients

2 chicken breasts

1 tbsp mayonnaise

2 eggs

1 tbsp chili pepper

1 tbsp curry powder

1 tbsp sugar

1 tbsp soy sauce

Directions

Put the chicken breasts on a clean flat surface and use a knife to slice in diagonal pieces. Gently pound them to become thinner using a rolling pin. Place in a bowl and add soy sauce, sugar, curry powder, and chili pepper.

Mix well and refrigerate for an hour; preheat the Air Fryer to 350 F. Remove the chicken and crack the eggs on. Add the mayonnaise and mix. Remove each chicken piece and shake well to remove as much liquid as possible.

Place them in the fryer basket and cook for 8 minutes. Flip and cook further for 6 minutes. Remove onto a serving platter and continue to cook with the remaining chicken. Serve with a side of steam greens.

209. Holiday Lemony Cornish Hen

Preparation Time: 14 hrs 20 minutes
Servings: 4

Ingredients

2 lb cornish hen

1 lemon, zested

¼ tbsp sugar

¼ tsp salt

1 tbsp chopped fresh rosemary

1 tbsp chopped fresh thyme

¼ tsp red pepper flakes

½ cup olive oil

Directions

Place the hen on a chopping board with its back facing you, and use a knife to cut through from the top of the backbone to the bottom of the backbone, making 2 cuts; remove the backbone. Divide the hen into two lengthwise while cutting through the breastplate; set aside.

In a bowl, add the lemon zest, sugar, salt, rosemary, thyme, red pepper flakes, and olive oil; mix well. Add the hen pieces, coat all around with the spoon, and place in the refrigerator to marinate for 14 hours.

Preheat the Air Fryer to 390 F. After the marinating time, remove the hen pieces from the marinade and pat dry with a paper towel. Place in the fryer basket and roast for 16 minutes. Remove to a platter and serve with veggies.

210. Italian Chicken Schnitzel with Herbs

Preparation Time: 25 minutes
Servings: 2

Ingredients

2 chicken breasts, skinless and boneless

2 eggs, cracked into a bowl

2 cups milk

4 tbsp tomato sauce

2 tbsp mixed herbs

2 cups mozzarella cheese

1 cup flour

¾ cup shaved ham

1 cup breadcrumbs

Directions

Place the chicken breast between to plastic wraps and use a rolling pin to pound them to flatten out. Whisk the milk and eggs together, in a bowl. Pour the flour in a plate, the breadcrumbs in another dish, and start coating the chicken. Toss the chicken in flour, then in the egg mixture, and then in the breadcrumbs.

Preheat the Air Fryer to 350 F. Put the chicken in the fryer basket and cook for 10 minutes. Remove them onto a plate and top the chicken with the ham, tomato sauce, mozzarella cheese, and mixed herbs. Return the chicken to the fryer's basket and cook further for 5 minutes or until the mozzarella cheese melts. Serve with vegetable fries.

211. Chicken with Honey and Orange

Preparation Time: 20 minutes
Servings: 4

Ingredients

1 ½ pounds chicken breast, washed and sliced

Parsley to taste

1 cup coconut, shredded

¾ cup breadcrumbs

2 whole eggs, beaten

½ cup flour

½ tsp pepper

Salt to taste

½ cup orange marmalade

1 tbsp red pepper flakes

¼ cup honey

3 tbsp Dijon mustard

Directions

Preheat your Air Fryer to 400 F. In a mixing bowl, combine coconut, flour, salt, parsley and pepper. In another bowl, add the beaten eggs. Place breadcrumbs in a third bowl. Dredge chicken in egg mix, flour and finally in the breadcrumbs. Place the chicken in the Air Fryer cooking basket and bake for 15 minutes.

In a separate bowl, mix honey, orange marmalade, mustard and pepper flakes. Cover chicken with marmalade mixture and fry for 5 more minutes. Enjoy!

212. Maple Turkey Breast with Sage

Preparation Time: 1 hour
Servings: 6

Ingredients

5 lb turkey breasts

¼ cup maple syrup

2 tbsp Dijon mustard

½ tbsp smoked paprika

1 tbsp thyme

2 tbsp olive oil

½ tbsp sage

½ tbsp salt and black pepper

1 tbsp butter, melted

Directions

Preheat the Air fryer to 350 F and brush the turkey with the olive oil. Combine all herbs and seasoning, in a small bowl, and rub the turkey with the mixture. Air fry the turkey for 25 minutes. Flip the turkey on its side and continue to cook for 12 more minutes.

Now, turn on the opposite side, and again, cook for an additional 12 minutes. Whisk the butter, maple and mustard together in a small bowl. When done, brush the glaze all over the turkey. Return to the air fryer and cook for 5 more minutes, until nice and crispy.

213. Parmesan Turkey Meatballs

Preparation Time: 40 minutes
Servings: 3 to 4

Ingredients

1 lb ground turkey

1 egg

½ cup breadcrumbs

1 tbsp garlic powder

1 tbsp Italian seasoning

1 tbsp onion powder

¼ cup Parmesan cheese, grated

Salt and black pepper to taste

Directions

Preheat the Air Fryer to 400 F. In a bowl, add the ground turkey, crack the egg onto it, add the breadcrumbs, garlic powder, onion powder, Italian seasoning, parmesan cheese, salt, and pepper. Use your hands to mix them well. Spoon out portions and make bite-size balls out of the mixture.

Grease the fryer basket with cooking spray and add 10 turkey balls to the fryer's basket; cook for 12 minutes. Slide out the fryer basket halfway through and shake. When ready, remove onto a serving platter and continue the cooking process for the remaining balls. Serve the turkey balls with marinara sauce and a side of noodles.

214. Chicken Wings with Parmesan and Oregano

Preparation Time: 35 minutes
Servings: 2

Ingredients

1 lb chicken wings

¼ cup butter

¼ cup grated Parmesan cheese

2 cloves garlic, minced

½ tbsp dried oregano

½ tbsp dried rosemary

Salt and black pepper to taste to season

¼ tsp paprika

Directions

Preheat the Air Fryer to 370 F. Place the chicken in a plate and season with salt and pepper. Put the chicken in the fryer basket, close the Air Fryer, and fry for 5 minutes. Meanwhile, place a skillet over medium heat on a stove top, add the butter, once melted add the garlic, stir and cook it for 1 minute.

Add the paprika, oregano, and rosemary to a bowl and mix them using a spoon. Add the mixture to the butter sauce. Stir and turn off the heat. Once the chicken breasts are ready, top them with the sauce, sprinkle with Parmesan cheese and cook in the Air Fryer for 5 minutes at 360 F.

215. Savory Chicken Breasts with Turmeric

Preparation Time: 20 minutes
Servings: 3

Ingredients

3 chicken breasts

Salt to season

¼ cup sweet chili sauce

3 tbsp turmeric

Directions

Preheat the Air Fryer to 390 F. In a bowl, add the salt, sweet chili sauce, and turmeric; mix evenly with a spoon. Place the chicken breasts on a clean flat surface and with a brush, apply the turmeric sauce lightly on the chicken. Place in the fryer basket and grill for 18 minutes; turn them halfway through.

216. Buttery Chicken Legs with Rice

Preparation Time: 40 minutes
Servings: 4

Ingredients

4 chicken legs

1 cup rice

2 cups water

2 tomatoes, cubed

3 tbsp butter

1 tbsp tomato paste

Salt and black pepper

1 onion

3 minced cloves garlic

Directions

Rub the chicken legs with butter. Sprinkle with salt and pepper and fry in a preheated Air Fryer for 30 minutes at 380 F. Then, add small onion and a little bit of oil; keep stirring. Add the tomatoes, the tomato paste, and the garlic, and cook for 5 more minutes.

Meanwhile, in a pan, boil the rice in 2 cups of water for around 20 minutes. In a baking tray, place the rice and top it with the air fried chicken and cook in the Air Fryer for 5 minutes. Serve and enjoy!

217. Chicken Thighs with Tomatoes

Preparation Time: 20 minutes
Servings: 2

Ingredients

2 chicken thighs

1 cup tomatoes, quartered

4 cloves garlic, minced

½ tbsp dried tarragon

½ tbsp olive oil

¼ tsp red pepper flakes

Salt and black pepper to taste

Directions

Preheat the Air Fryer to 390 F. Add the tomatoes, red pepper flakes, tarragon, garlic, and olive oil to a medium bowl. Use a spoon to mix well. In a large ramekin, add the chicken and top with the tomato mixture.

Place the ramekin in the fryer basket and roast for 10 minutes. After baking, carefully remove the ramekin. Plate the chicken thighs, spoon the cooking juice over and serve.

218. Spicy Black Beans with Chicken and Corn

Preparation Time: 18 minutes
Servings: 4

Ingredients

4 boneless and skinless chicken breasts, cubed

1 can sweet corn

1 can black beans, rinsed and drained

1 cup red and green peppers, stripes, cooked

1 tbsp vegetable oil

2 tbsp chili powder

Directions

Coat the chicken with salt, black pepper and a sprinkle of oil; cook for 15 minutes at 380 F. Meanwhile, in a deep skillet, pour 1 tbsp. of oil and stir in the chili powder, the corn and the beans. Add a little bit of hot water and keep stirring for 3 more minutes. Transfer the corn, the beans and the chicken to a serving platter. Enjoy.

219. Spicy Yogurt Chicken Strips

Preparation Time: 25 minutes
Servings: 4

Ingredients

1 cup breadcrumbs

½ cup yogurt

1 lb chicken breasts cut into strips

1 tbsp ground cayenne

1 tbsp hot sauce

2 beaten eggs

1 tbsp sweet paprika

1 tbsp garlic powder

Directions

Preheat the air fryer to 390 degrees F. Whisk the eggs along with the hot sauce and yogurt. In a shallow bowl, combine the breadcrumbs, paprika, pepper, and garlic powder. Line a baking dish with parchment paper.

Dip the chicken in the egg/yogurt mixture first, and then coat with breadcrumbs. Arrange on the sheet and bake in the air fryer for 8 minutes. Flip the chicken over and bake for 8 more minutes on the other side.

220. Crispy Cajun Chicken Tenders

Preparation Time: 25 minutes
Servings: 4

Ingredients

3 lb chicken breast cut into slices

3 eggs

2 ¼ cup flour, divided

1 tbsp olive oil

½ tbsp plus

½ tbsp garlic powder, divided

1 tbsp salt

3 tbsp cajun seasoning, divided

¼ cup milk

Directions

Season the chicken with salt, pepper, ½ tbsp garlic powder and 2 tbsp Cajun seasoning.

Combine 2 cups flour, the rest of the Cajun seasoning and the rest of the garlic powder, in a bowl. In another bowl, whisk the eggs, milk, olive oil, and quarter cup flour. Preheat the Air fryer to 370 F.

Line a baking sheet with parchment paper. Dip the chicken into the egg mixture first, and then into the flour mixture. Arrange on the sheet. If there isn't enough room, work in two batches. Cook for 12 to 15 minutes.

221. Fried Chicken Tenderloins

Preparation Time: 15 minutes
Servings: 4

Ingredients

8 chicken tenderloins

2 tbsp butter

2 oz breadcrumbs

1 large egg, whisked

Directions

Preheat the Air fryer to 380 F. Combine the butter and the breadcrumbs, in a bowl. Keep mixing and stirring until the mixture gets crumbly. Dip the chicken in the egg wash. Then dip the chicken in the crumbs mix.

Making sure it is evenly and fully covered; cook for 10 minutes. Serve the dish and enjoy its crispy taste!

222. Parmesan Chicken Fingers with Fresh Chives

Preparation Time: 8 minutes
Servings: 2

Ingredients

2 medium-sized chicken breasts, cut in stripes

3 tbsp Parmesan cheese, grated

¼ tbsp fresh chives, chopped

⅓ cup breadcrumbs

1 egg white

2 tbsp plum sauce, optional

½ tbsp fresh thyme, chopped

½ tbsp black pepper

1 tbsp water

Directions

Preheat the Air Fryer to 360 F. Mix the chives, Parmesan cheese, thyme, pepper and breadcrumbs. In another bowl, whisk the egg white and mix with the water. Dip the chicken strips into the egg mixture and the breadcrumb mixture. Place the strips in the air fryer basket and cook for 10 minutes. Serve with plum sauce.

223. Mom's Tarragon Chicken Breasts

Preparation Time: 15 minutes
Servings: 3

Ingredients

1 boneless and skinless chicken breast

½ tbsp butter

¼ tbsp kosher salt

¼ cup dried tarragon

¼ tbsp black and fresh ground pepper

Directions

Preheat the Air Fryer to 380 F and place each chicken breast on a 12x12 inches foil wrap. Top the chicken with tarragon and butter; season with salt and pepper to taste. Wrap the foil around the chicken breast in a loose way to create a flow of air. Cook the in the Air Fryer for 15 minutes. Carefully unwrap the chicken and serve.

224. Creamy Chicken and Ham

Preparation Time: 40 minutes
Servings: 4

Ingredients

4 skinless and boneless chicken breasts

4 slices ham

4 slices Swiss cheese

3 tbsp all-purpose flour

4 tbsp butter

1 tbsp paprika

1 tbsp chicken bouillon granules

½ cup dry white wine

1 cup heavy whipping cream

1 tbsp cornstarch

Directions

Preheat the Air Fryer to 380 F. Pound the chicken breasts and put a slice of ham on each of the chicken breasts. Fold the edges of the chicken over the filling and secure the edges with toothpicks. In a medium bowl, combine the paprika and the flour, and coat the chicken pieces. Fry the chicken for 20 minutes.

In a large skillet, heat the butter and add the bouillon and wine; reduce the heat to low. Remove the chicken from the Air Fryer and place it in the skillet. Let simmer for around 20-25 minutes.

225. Stuffed Turkey Brestas with Ham, Cheese and Herbs

Preparation Time: 35 minutes
Servings: 4

Ingredients

2 turkey breasts

1 ham slice

1 slice cheddar cheese

2 oz breadcrumbs

1 tbsp cream cheese

1 tbsp garlic powder

1 tbsp thyme

1 tbsp tarragon

1 egg, beaten

Salt and black pepper to taste

Directions

Preheat the air fryer to 350 F. Cut the turkey in the middle, that way so you can add ingredients in the center. Season with salt, pepper, thyme and tarragon. Combine the cream cheese and garlic powder, in a small bowl.

Spread the mixture on the inside of the breasts. Place half cheddar slice and half ham slice in the center of each breast. Dip the cordon bleu in egg first, then sprinkle with breadcrumbs. Cook on a baking mat for 30 minutes.

226. Cayenne Cauliflower Florets with Chicken Drumsticks

Preparation Time: 50 minutes
Servings: 4

Ingredients

8 chicken drumsticks

2 tbsp oregano

2 tbsp thyme

2 oz oats

¼ cup milk

¼ steamed cauliflower florets

1 egg

1 tbsp ground cayenne

Salt and black pepper to taste

Directions

Preheat the Air fryer to 350 F and season the drumsticks with salt and pepper; rub them with the milk. Place all the other ingredients, except the egg, in a food processor. Process until smooth. Dip each drumstick in the egg first, and then in the oat mixture. Arrange half of them on a baking mat inside the air fryer. Cook for 20 minutes. Repeat with the other batch.

227. Party Hot Chicken Wings

Preparation Time: 4 hrs 20 minutes
Servings: 2

Ingredients

8 chicken wings

1 tbsp water

2 tbsp potato starch

2 tbsp cornstarch

2 tbsp hot curry paste

½ tbsp baking powder

Directions

Combine the hot curry paste and water, in a small bowl. Place the wings in a large bowl, add the tom yum mixture and coat well. Cover the bowl and refrigerate for 4 hours. Preheat the air fryer to 370 degrees.

Combine the baking powder, cornstarch and potato starch. Dip each wing in the starch mixture. Place on a lined baking dish in the air fryer and cook for 7 minutes. Flip over and cook for 5 to 7 minutes more.

228. Oregano Chicken Legs with Lemon

Preparation Time: 50 minutes
Servings: 5

Ingredients

5 quarters chicken legs

2 lemons, halved

5 tbsp garlic powder

5 tbsp dried basil

5 tbsp oregano, dried

⅓ cup olive oil

Salt and black pepper

Directions

Set the Air Fryer to 350 F. Place the chicken in a large deep bowl. Brush the chicken legs with a tbsp of olive oil.

Sprinkle with the lemon juice and arrange in the Air Fryer. In another bowl, combine basil, oregano, garlic powder, salt and pepper. Sprinkle the seasoning mixture on the chicken. Cook in the preheated Air Fryer for 50 minutes, shaking every 10-15 minutes.

229. Chicken with Cashew Nuts and Bell Pepper

Preparation Time: 30 minutes
Servings: 4

Ingredients

1 lb chicken cubes

2 tbsp soy sauce

1 tbsp corn flour

2 ½ onion cubes

1 carrot, chopped

⅓ cup cashew nuts, fried

1 bell pepper, cut

2 tbsp garlic, crushed

Salt and white pepper

Directions

Marinate the chicken cubes with ½ tbsp of white pepper, ½ tsp salt, 2 tbsp soya sauce, and add 1 tbsp corn flour.

Set aside for 25 minutes. Preheat the Air Fryer to 380 F and transfer the marinated chicken. Add the garlic, the onion, the bell pepper, and the carrot; fry for 5-6 minutes. Roll it in the cashew nuts before serving.

230. Oyster Chicken Breasts

Preparation Time: 60 minutes
Servings: 2

Ingredients

2 chicken breasts

1 tbsp minced ginger

2 rosemary sprigs

½ lemon, cut into wedges

1 tbsp soy sauce

½ tbsp olive oil

1 tbsp oyster sauce

3 tbsp brown sugar

Directions

Add the ginger, soy sauce, and olive oil, in a bowl; add the chicken and coat well. Cover the bowl and refrigerate for 30 minutes. Preheat the air fryer to 370 F. Transfer the marinated chicken to a baking dish; cook for 6 minutes.

Meanwhile, mix the oyster sauce, rosemary and brown sugar, in a small bowl. Pour the sauce over the chicken. Arrange the lemon wedges in the dish. Return to the air fryer and cook for

Chapter 7. Vegan and vegetarian recipes

231. Cauliflower Steak

Preparation Time: 12 minutes
Servings: 4

Ingredients:

1 medium head cauliflower

¼ cup blue cheese crumbles

¼ cup hot sauce

¼ cup full-fat ranch dressing

2 tbsp. salted butter; melted.

Directions:

Remove cauliflower leaves. Slice the head in ½-inch-thick slices.

In a small bowl, mix hot sauce and butter. Brush the mixture over the cauliflower.

Place each cauliflower steak into the air fryer, working in batches if necessary. Adjust the temperature to 400 Degrees F and set the timer for 7 minutes

When cooked, edges will begin turning dark and caramelized. To serve, sprinkle steaks with crumbled blue cheese. Drizzle with ranch dressing.

Nutrition: Calories: 122; Protein: 4.9g; Fiber: 3.0g; Fat: 8.4g; Carbs: 7.7g

232. Chocolate Chip Pan Cookie

Preparation Time: 17 minutes
Servings: 4

Ingredients:

½ cup blanched finely ground almond flour.

1 large egg.

¼ cup powdered erythritol

2 tbsp. unsalted butter; softened.

2 tbsp. low-carb, sugar-free chocolate chips

½ tsp. unflavored gelatin

½ tsp. baking powder.

½ tsp. vanilla extract.

Directions:

Take a large bowl, mix almond flour and erythritol. Stir in butter, egg and gelatin until combined.

Stir in baking powder and vanilla and then fold in chocolate chips

Pour batter into 6-inch round baking pan. Place pan into the air fryer basket.

Adjust the temperature to 300 Degrees F and set the timer for 7 minutes

When fully cooked, the top will be golden brown and a toothpick inserted in center will come out clean. Let cool at least 10 minutes.

Nutrition: Calories: 188; Protein: 5.6g; Fiber: 2.0g; Fat: 15.7g; Carbs: 16.8g

233. Mustard Greens and Green Beans

Preparation Time: 22 minutes
Servings: 4

Ingredients:

1 lb. green beans; halved

¼ cup tomato puree

3 garlic cloves; minced

1 bunch mustard greens, trimmed

2 tbsp. olive oil

1 tbsp. balsamic vinegar

Salt and black pepper to taste.

Directions:

In a pan that fits your air fryer, mix the mustard greens with the rest of the ingredients, toss, put the pan in the fryer and cook at 350°F for 12 minutes

Divide everything between plates and serve.

Nutrition: Calories: 163; Fat: 4g; Fiber: 3g; Carbs: 4g; Protein: 7g

234. Artichoke Spinach Casserole

Preparation Time: 30 minutes
Servings: 4

Ingredients:

⅓ cup full-fat mayonnaise

8 oz. full-fat cream cheese; softened.

¼ cup diced yellow onion

⅓ cup full-fat sour cream.

¼ cup chopped pickled jalapeños.

2 cups fresh spinach; chopped

2 cups cauliflower florets; chopped

1 cup artichoke hearts; chopped

1 tbsp. salted butter; melted.

Directions:

Take a large bowl, mix butter, onion, cream cheese, mayonnaise and sour cream. Fold in jalapeños, spinach, cauliflower and artichokes.

Pour the mixture into a 4-cup round baking dish. Cover with foil and place into the air fryer basket

Adjust the temperature to 370 Degrees F and set the timer for 15 minutes. In the last 2 minutes of cooking, remove the foil to brown the top. Serve warm.

Nutrition: Calories: 423; Protein: 6.7g; Fiber: 5.3g; Fat: 36.3g; Carbs: 12.1g

235. Baked Egg and Veggies

Preparation Time: 20 minutes
Servings: 2

Ingredients:

1 cup fresh spinach; chopped

1 small zucchini, sliced lengthwise and quartered

1 medium Roma tomato; diced

½ medium green bell pepper; seeded and diced

2 large eggs.

2 tbsp. salted butter

¼ tsp. garlic powder.

¼ tsp. onion powder.

½ tsp. dried basil

¼ tsp. dried oregano.

Directions:

Grease two (4-inchramekins with 1 tbsp. butter each.

Take a large bowl, toss zucchini, bell pepper, spinach and tomatoes. Divide the mixture in two and place half in each ramekin.

Crack an egg on top of each ramekin and sprinkle with onion powder, garlic powder, basil and oregano. Place into the air fryer basket. Adjust the temperature to 330 Degrees F and set the timer for 10 minutes. Serve immediately.

Nutrition: Calories: 150; Protein: 8.3g; Fiber: 2.2g; Fat: 10.0g; Carbs: 6.6g

236. Mini Cheesecake

Preparation Time: 25 minutes
Servings: 2

Ingredients:

4 oz. full-fat cream cheese; softened.

⅛ cup powdered erythritol

1 large egg.

½ cup walnuts

2 tbsp. granular erythritol.

2 tbsp. salted butter

½ tsp. vanilla extract.

Directions:

Place walnuts, butter and granular erythritol in a food processor. Pulse until ingredients stick together and a dough forms

Press dough into 4-inch springform pan then place the pan into the air fryer basket.

Adjust the temperature to 400 Degrees F and set the timer for 5 minutes. When timer beeps, remove the crust and let cool

Take a medium bowl, mix cream cheese with egg, vanilla extract and powdered erythritol until smooth.

Spoon mixture on top of baked walnut crust and place into the air fryer basket. Adjust the temperature to 300 Degrees F and set the timer for 10 minutes. Once done, chill for 2 hours before serving

Nutrition: Calories: 531; Protein: 11.4g; Fiber: 2.3g; Fat: 48.3g; Carbs: 31.4g

237. Savoy Cabbage

Preparation Time: 20 minutes
Servings: 4

Ingredients:

1 Savoy cabbage head, shredded

1 tbsp. dill; chopped.

1 ½ tbsp. ghee; melted

¼ cup coconut cream

Salt and black pepper to taste.

Directions:

In a pan that fits the air fryer, combine all the ingredients except the coconut cream, toss, put the pan in the air fryer and cook at 390°F for 10 minutes

Add the cream, toss, cook for 5 minutes more, divide between plates and serve

Nutrition: Calories: 173; Fat: 5g; Fiber: 3g; Carbs: 5g; Protein: 8g

238. Spaghetti Squash Alfredo.

Preparation Time: 25 minutes
Servings: 2

Ingredients:

½ large cooked spaghetti squash

¼ cup grated vegetarian Parmesan cheese.

½ cup shredded Italian blend cheese

½ cup low-carb Alfredo sauce

2 tbsp. salted butter; melted.

¼ tsp. ground peppercorn

½ tsp. garlic powder.

1 tsp. dried parsley.

Directions:

Using a fork, remove the strands of spaghetti squash from the shell. Place into a large bowl with butter and Alfredo sauce. Sprinkle with Parmesan, garlic powder, parsley and peppercorn

Pour into a 4-cup round baking dish and top with shredded cheese. Place dish into the air fryer basket. Adjust the temperature to 320 Degrees F and set the timer for 15 minutes.

When finished, cheese will be golden and bubbling. Serve immediately

Nutrition: Calories: 375; Protein: 13.5g; Fiber: 4.0g; Fat: 24.2g; Carbs: 24.1g

239. Vanilla Pound Cake.

Preparation Time: 35 minutes
Servings: 6

Ingredients:

½ cup full-fat sour cream.

1 oz. full-fat cream cheese; softened.

2 large eggs.

½ cup granular erythritol.

1 cup blanched finely ground almond flour.

¼ cup salted butter; melted.

1 tsp. baking powder.

1 tsp. vanilla extract.

Directions:

Take a large bowl, mix almond flour, butter and erythritol.

Add in vanilla, baking powder, sour cream and cream cheese and mix until well combined. Add eggs and mix.

Pour batter into a 6-inch round baking pan. Place pan into the air fryer basket. Adjust the temperature to 300 Degrees F and set the timer for 25 minutes.

When the cake is done, a toothpick inserted in center will come out clean. The center should not feel wet. Allow it to cool completely, or the cake will crumble when moved.

Nutrition: Calories: 253; Protein: 6.9g; Fiber: 2.0g; Fat: 22.6g; Carbs: 25.2g

240. Pumpkin Spice Pecans

Preparation Time: 11 minutes
Servings: 4

Ingredients:

1 cup whole pecans

1 large egg. white

¼ cup granular erythritol.

½ tsp. pumpkin pie spice

½ tsp. vanilla extract.

½ tsp. ground cinnamon.

Directions:

Toss all ingredients in a large bowl until pecans are coated. Place into the air fryer basket.

Adjust the temperature to 300 Degrees F and set the timer for 6 minutes. Toss two to three times during cooking. Allow to cool completely. Store in an airtight container up to 3 days

Nutrition: Calories: 178; Protein: 3.2g; Fiber: 2.6g; Fat: 17.0g; Carbs: 19.0g

241. Cream Puffs

Preparation Time: 21 minutes
Servings: 8 puffs

Ingredients:

2 oz. full-fat cream cheese.

1 large egg.

¼ cup powdered erythritol

½ cup blanched finely ground almond flour.

½ cup low-carb vanilla protein powder

½ cup granular erythritol.

2 tbsp. heavy whipping cream.

5 tbsp. unsalted butter; melted.

½ tsp. baking powder.

¼ tsp. ground cinnamon.

½ tsp. vanilla extract.

Directions:

Mix almond flour, protein powder, granular erythritol, baking powder, egg and butter in a large bowl until a soft dough forms.

Place the dough in the freezer for 20 minutes. Wet your hands with water and roll the dough into eight balls.

Cut a piece of parchment to fit your air fryer basket. Working in batches as necessary, place the dough balls into the air fryer basket on top of parchment.

Adjust the temperature to 380 Degrees F and set the timer for 6 minutes. Flip cream puffs halfway through the cooking time.

When the timer beeps, remove the puffs and allow to cool.

Take a medium bowl, beat the cream cheese, powdered erythritol, cinnamon, cream and vanilla until fluffy.

Place the mixture into a pastry bag or a storage bag with the end snipped. Cut a small hole in the bottom of each puff and fill with some of the cream mixture. Store in an airtight container up to 2 days in the refrigerator.

Nutrition: Calories: 178; Protein: 14.9g; Fiber: 1.3g; Fat: 12.1g; Carbs: 22.1g

242. Tomato and Asparagus

Preparation Time: 20 minutes
Servings: 4

Ingredients:

1 lb. asparagus, trimmed

1 jalapeno pepper; chopped.

10 cherry tomatoes; halved

2 green onions; chopped.

1 tbsp. olive oil

2 tsp. chili powder

A pinch of salt and black pepper

Directions:

In a pan that fits your air fryer, mix the asparagus with tomatoes and the rest of the ingredients, toss.

Put the pan in the fryer and cook at 390°F for 15 minutes

Divide the mix between plates and serve.

Nutrition: Calories: 173; Fat: 4g; Fiber: 2g; Carbs: 4g; Protein: 6g

243. Peanut Butter Cheesecake Brownies

Preparation Time: 55 minutes
Servings: 6

Ingredients:

½ cup blanched finely ground almond flour.

8 oz. full-fat cream cheese; softened.

¼ cup unsalted butter; softened.

2 large eggs, divided.

1 cup powdered erythritol, divided.

¼ cup heavy whipping cream.

2 tbsp. unsweetened cocoa powder

½ tsp. baking powder.

2 tbsp. no-sugar-added peanut butter

1 tsp. vanilla extract.

Directions:

Take a large bowl, mix almond flour, ½ cup erythritol, cocoa powder and baking powder. Stir in butter and one egg.

Scoop mixture into 6-inch round baking pan. Place pan into the air fryer basket. Adjust the temperature to 300 Degrees F and set the timer for 20 minutes.

When fully cooked a toothpick inserted in center will come out clean. Allow 20 minutes to fully cool and firm up

Take a large bowl, beat cream cheese, remaining ½ cup erythritol, heavy cream, vanilla, peanut butter and remaining egg until fluffy.

Pour mixture over cooled brownies. Place pan back into the air fryer basket. Adjust the temperature to 300 Degrees F and set the timer for 15 minutes

Cheesecake will be slightly browned and mostly firm with a slight jiggle when done.

Allow to cool, then refrigerate 2 hours before serving.

Nutrition: Calories: 347; Protein: 8.3g; Fiber: 2.0g; Fat: 30.9g; Carbs: 29.8g

244. BBQ Pulled Mushrooms

Preparation Time: 17 minutes
Servings: 2

Ingredients:

4 large portobello mushrooms

½ cup low-carb, sugar-free barbecue sauce

1 tbsp. salted butter; melted.

1 tsp. paprika

¼ tsp. onion powder.

¼ tsp. ground black pepper

1 tsp. chili powder

Directions:

Remove stem and scoop out the underside of each mushroom. Brush the caps with butter and sprinkle with pepper, chili powder, paprika and onion powder.

Place mushrooms into the air fryer basket. Adjust the temperature to 400 Degrees F and set the timer for 8 minutes.

When the timer beeps, remove mushrooms from the basket and place on a cutting board or work surface. Using two forks, gently pull the mushrooms apart, creating strands.

Place mushroom strands into a 4-cup round baking dish with barbecue sauce. Place dish into the air fryer basket.

Adjust the temperature to 350 Degrees F and set the timer for 4 minutes. Stir halfway through the cooking time. Serve warm.

Nutrition: Calories: 108; Protein: 3.3g; Fiber: 2.7g; Fat: 5.9g; Carbs: 10.9g

245. Blackberry Crisp

Preparation Time: 20 minutes
Servings: 4

Ingredients:

1 cup Crunchy Granola

2 cups blackberries

⅓ cup powdered erythritol

2 tbsp. lemon juice

¼ tsp. xanthan gum

Directions:

Take a large bowl, toss blackberries, erythritol, lemon juice and xanthan gum.

Pour into 6-inch round baking dish and cover with foil. Place into the air fryer basket.

Adjust the temperature to 350 Degrees F and set the timer for 12 minutes.

When the timer beeps, remove the foil and stir.

Sprinkle granola over mixture and return to the air fryer basket. Adjust the temperature to 320 Degrees F and set the timer for 3 minutes or until top is golden. Serve warm.

Nutrition: Calories: 496; Protein: 9.2g; Fiber: 12.5g; Fat: 42.1g; Carbs: 44.0g

246. Cheese Zucchini Boats

Preparation Time: 35 minutes
Servings: 2

Ingredients:

2 medium zucchini

¼ cup full-fat ricotta cheese

¼ cup shredded mozzarella cheese

¼ cup low-carb, no-sugar-added pasta sauce.

2 tbsp. grated vegetarian Parmesan cheese

1 tbsp. avocado oil

¼ tsp. garlic powder.

½ tsp. dried parsley.

¼ tsp. dried oregano.

Directions:

Cut off 1-inch from the top and bottom of each zucchini.

Slice zucchini in half lengthwise and use a spoon to scoop out a bit of the inside, making room for filling. Brush with oil and spoon 2 tbsp. pasta sauce into each shell

Take a medium bowl, mix ricotta, mozzarella, oregano, garlic powder and parsley

Spoon the mixture into each zucchini shell. Place stuffed zucchini shells into the air fryer basket.

Adjust the temperature to 350 Degrees F and set the timer for 20 minutes

To remove from the fryer basket, use tongs or a spatula and carefully lift out. Top with Parmesan. Serve immediately.

Nutrition: Calories: 215; Protein: 10.5g; Fiber: 2.7g; Fat: 14.9g; Carbs: 9.3g

247. Green Beans and Lime Sauce

Preparation Time: 13 minutes
Servings: 4

Ingredients:

1 lb. green beans, trimmed

2 tbsp. ghee; melted

1 tbsp. lime juice

1 tsp. chili powder

A pinch of salt and black pepper

Directions:

Take a bowl and mix the ghee with the rest of the ingredients except the green beans and whisk really well.

Mix the green beans with the lime sauce, toss

Put them in your air fryer's basket and cook at 400°F for 8 minutes. Serve right away.

Nutrition: Calories: 151; Fat: 4g; Fiber: 2g; Carbs: 4g; Protein: 6g

248. Roasted Broccoli Salad

Preparation Time: 17 minutes
Servings: 2

Ingredients:

3 cups fresh broccoli florets.

½ medium lemon.

¼ cup sliced almonds.

2 tbsp. salted butter; melted.

Directions:

Place broccoli into a 6-inch round baking dish. Pour butter over broccoli. Add almonds and toss. Place dish into the air fryer basket

Adjust the temperature to 380 Degrees F and set the timer for 7 minutes. Stir halfway through the cooking time. When timer beeps, zest lemon onto broccoli and squeeze juice into pan. Toss. Serve warm.

Nutrition: Calories: 215; Protein: 6.4g; Fiber: 5.0g; Fat: 16.3g; Carbs: 12.1g

249. Quiche Stuffed Peppers

Preparation Time: 20 minutes
Servings: 2

Ingredients:

2 medium green bell peppers

3 large eggs.

½ cup chopped broccoli

½ cup shredded medium Cheddar cheese.

¼ cup diced yellow onion

¼ cup full-fat ricotta cheese

Directions:

Cut the tops off of the peppers and remove the seeds and white membranes with a small knife. Take a medium bowl, whisk eggs and ricotta

Add onion and broccoli. Pour the egg and vegetable mixture evenly into each pepper. Top with Cheddar. Place peppers into a 4-cup round baking dish and place into the air fryer basket. Adjust the temperature to 350 Degrees F and set the timer for 15 minutes

Eggs will be mostly firm and peppers tender when fully cooked. Serve immediately.

Nutrition: Calories: 314; Protein: 21.6g; Fiber: 3.0g; Fat: 18.7g; Carbs: 10.8g

250. Monkey Bread

Preparation Time: 27 minutes
Servings: 6

Ingredients:

½ cup blanched finely ground almond flour.

1 oz. full-fat cream cheese; softened.

1 large egg.

¼ cup heavy whipping cream.

½ cup low-carb vanilla protein powder

¾ cup granular erythritol, divided

8 tbsp. salted butter; melted and divided

½ tsp. vanilla extract.

½ tsp. baking powder

Directions:

Take a large bowl, combine almond flour, protein powder, ½ cup erythritol, baking powder, 5 tbsp. butter, cream cheese and egg. A soft, sticky dough will form.

Place the dough in the freezer for 20 minutes. It will be firm enough to roll into balls. Wet your hands with warm water and roll into twelve balls. Place the balls into a 6-inch round baking dish

In a medium skillet over medium heat, melt remaining butter with remaining erythritol. Lower the heat and continue stirring until mixture turns golden, then add cream and vanilla. Remove from heat and allow it to thicken for a few minutes while you continue to stir

While the mixture cools, place baking dish into the air fryer basket. Adjust the temperature to 320 Degrees F and set the timer for 6 minutes

When the timer beeps, flip the monkey bread over onto a plate and slide it back into the baking pan. Cook an additional 4 minutes until all the tops are brown.

Pour the caramel sauce over the monkey bread and cook an additional 2 minutes.

Let cool completely before serving.

Nutrition: Calories: 322; Protein: 20.4g; Fiber: 1.7g; Fat: 24.5g; Carbs: 33.7g

251. Broccoli Crust Pizza

Preparation Time: 27 minutes
Servings: 4

Ingredients:

3 cups riced broccoli, steamed and drained well

½ cup shredded mozzarella cheese

½ cup grated vegetarian Parmesan cheese.

1 large egg.

3 tbsp. low-carb Alfredo sauce

Directions:

Take a large bowl, mix broccoli, egg and Parmesan.

Cut a piece of parchment to fit your air fryer basket. Press out the pizza mixture to fit on the parchment, working in two batches if necessary. Place into the air fryer basket. Adjust the temperature to 370 Degrees F and set the timer for 5 minutes.

When the timer beeps, the crust should be firm enough to flip. If not, add 2 additional minutes. Flip crust.

Top with Alfredo sauce and mozzarella. Return to the air fryer basket and cook an additional 7 minutes or until cheese is golden and bubbling. Serve warm.

Nutrition: Calories: 136; Protein: 9.9g; Fiber: 2.3g; Fat: 7.6g; Carbs:5.7g

252. Cheesy Zoodle Bake

Preparation Time: 18 minutes
Servings: 4

Ingredients:

½ cup heavy whipping cream.

2 oz. full-fat cream cheese.

1 cup shredded sharp Cheddar cheese.

2 medium zucchini, spiralized

¼ cup diced white onion

2 tbsp. salted butter

½ tsp. minced garlic

Directions:

In a large saucepan over medium heat, melt butter. Add onion and sauté until it begins to soften, 1–3 minutes. Add garlic and sauté 30 seconds, then pour in cream and add cream cheese

Remove the pan from heat and stir in Cheddar. Add the zucchini and toss in the sauce, then put into a 4-cup round baking dish.

Cover the dish with foil and place into the air fryer basket. Adjust the temperature to 370 Degrees F and set the timer for 8 minutes

After 6 minutes remove the foil and let the top brown for remaining cooking time. Stir and serve.

Nutrition: Calories: 337; Protein: 9.6g; Fiber: 1.2g; Fat: 28.4g; Carbs: 5.9g

253. Eggplant Stacks

Preparation Time: 17 minutes
Servings: 4

Ingredients:

2 large tomatoes; cut into ¼-inch slices

¼ cup fresh basil, sliced

4 oz. fresh mozzarella; cut into ½-oz. slices

1 medium eggplant; cut into ¼-inch slices

2 tbsp. olive oil

Directions:

In a 6-inch round baking dish, place four slices of eggplant on the bottom. Place a slice of tomato on top of each eggplant round, then mozzarella, then eggplant. Repeat as necessary.

Drizzle with olive oil. Cover dish with foil and place dish into the air fryer basket. Adjust the temperature to 350 Degrees F and set the timer for 12 minutes.

When done, eggplant will be tender. Garnish with fresh basil to serve.

Nutrition: Calories: 195; Protein: 8.5g; Fiber: 5.2g; Fat: 12.7g; Carbs: 12.7g

254. Roasted Garlic Zucchini Rolls

Preparation Time: 40 minutes
Servings: 4

Ingredients:

2 medium zucchini

½ cup full-fat ricotta cheese

¼ white onion; peeled.and diced

2 cups spinach; chopped

¼ cup heavy cream

½ cup sliced baby portobello mushrooms

¾ cup shredded mozzarella cheese, divided.

2 tbsp. unsalted butter.

2 tbsp. vegetable broth.

½ tsp. finely minced roasted garlic

¼ tsp. dried oregano.

⅛ tsp. xanthan gum

¼ tsp. salt

½ tsp. garlic powder.

Directions:

1 Using a mandoline or sharp knife, slice zucchini into long strips lengthwise. Place strips between paper towels to absorb moisture. Set aside

2 In a medium saucepan over medium heat, melt butter. Add onion and sauté until fragrant. Add garlic and sauté 30 seconds.

3 Pour in heavy cream, broth and xanthan gum. Turn off heat and whisk mixture until it begins to thicken, about 3 minutes.

4 Take a medium bowl, add ricotta, salt, garlic powder and oregano and mix well. Fold in spinach, mushrooms and ½ cup mozzarella

5 Pour half of the sauce into a 6-inch round baking pan. To assemble the rolls, place two strips of zucchini on a work surface. Spoon 2 tbsp. of ricotta mixture onto the slices and roll up. Place seam side down on top of sauce. Repeat with remaining ingredients

6 Pour remaining sauce over the rolls and sprinkle with remaining mozzarella. Cover with foil and place into the air fryer basket. Adjust the temperature to 350 Degrees F and set the timer for 20 minutes. In the last 5 minutes, remove the foil to brown the cheese. Serve immediately.

Nutrition: Calories: 245; Protein: 10.5g; Fiber: 1.8g; Fat: 18.9g; Carbs: 7.1g

255. Roasted Veggie Bowl

Preparation Time: 25 minutes
Servings: 2

Ingredients:

¼ medium white onion; peeled.and sliced ¼-inch thick

½ medium green bell pepper; seeded and sliced ¼-inch thick

1 cup broccoli florets

1 cup quartered Brussels sprouts

½ cup cauliflower florets

1 tbsp. coconut oil

½ tsp. garlic powder.

½ tsp. cumin

2 tsp. chili powder

Directions:

Toss all ingredients together in a large bowl until vegetables are fully coated with oil and seasoning. Pour vegetables into the air fryer basket.

Adjust the temperature to 360 Degrees F and set the timer for 15 minutes. Shake two or three times during cooking. Serve warm.

Nutrition: Calories: 121; Protein: 4.3g; Fiber: 5.2g; Fat: 7.1g; Carbs: 13.1g

256. Espresso Mini Cheesecake

Preparation Time: 20 minutes
Servings: 2

Ingredients:

½ cup walnuts

4 oz. full-fat cream cheese; softened.

1 large egg.

2 tbsp. salted butter

2 tbsp. granular erythritol.

2 tbsp. powdered erythritol

1 tsp. espresso powder

½ tsp. vanilla extract.

2 tsp. unsweetened cocoa powder

Directions:

Place walnuts, butter and granular erythritol in a food processor. Pulse until ingredients stick together and a dough forms.

Press dough into 4-inch springform pan and place into the air fryer basket.

Adjust the temperature to 400 Degrees F and set the timer for 5 minutes. When timer beeps, remove crust and let cool.

Take a medium bowl, mix cream cheese with egg, vanilla extract, powdered erythritol, cocoa powder and espresso powder until smooth.

Spoon mixture on top of baked walnut crust and place into the air fryer basket. Adjust the temperature for 300 Degrees F and set the timer for 10 minutes. Once done, chill for 2 hours before serving.

Nutrition: Calories: 535; Protein: 11.6g; Fiber: 7.2g; Fat: 48.4g; Carbs: 37.1g

257. Bacon Snack

Preparation Time: 15 minutes
Servings: 4

Ingredients:

1 cup dark chocolate; melted

4 bacon slices; halved

A pinch of pink salt

Directions:

Dip each bacon slice in some chocolate, sprinkle pink salt over them.

Put them in your air fryer's basket and cook at 350°F for 10 minutes

Nutrition: Calories: 151; Fat: 4g; Fiber: 2g; Carbs: 4g; Protein: 8g

258. Shrimp Snack

Preparation Time: 15 minutes
Servings: 4

Ingredients:

1 lb. shrimp; peeled and deveined

¼ cup olive oil

3 garlic cloves; minced

¼ tsp. cayenne pepper

Juice of ½ lemon

A pinch of salt and black pepper

Directions:

In a pan that fits your air fryer, mix all the ingredients, toss,

Introduce in the fryer and cook at 370°F for 10 minutes. Serve as a snack

Nutrition: Calories: 242; Fat: 14g; Fiber: 2g; Carbs: 3g; Protein: 17g

259. Avocado Wraps

Preparation Time: 20 minutes
Servings: 4

Ingredients:

2 avocados, peeled, pitted and cut into 12 wedges

1 tbsp. ghee; melted

12 bacon strips

Directions:

Wrap each avocado wedge in a bacon strip, brush them with the ghee.

Put them in your air fryer's basket and cook at 360°F for 15 minutes. Serve as an appetizer

Nutrition: Calories: 161; Fat: 4g; Fiber: 2g; Carbs: 4g; Protein: 6g

260. Cheesy Meatballs

Preparation Time: 30 minutes
Servings: 16 meatballs

Ingredients:

1 lb. 80/20 ground beef.

3 oz. low-moisture, whole-milk mozzarella, cubed

1 large egg.

½ cup low-carb, no-sugar-added pasta sauce.

¼ cup grated Parmesan cheese.

¼ cup blanched finely ground almond flour.

¼ tsp. onion powder.

1 tsp. dried parsley.

½ tsp. garlic powder.

Directions:

Take a large bowl, add ground beef, almond flour, parsley, garlic powder, onion powder and egg. Fold ingredients together until fully combined

Form the mixture into 2-inch balls and use your thumb or a spoon to create an indent in the center of each meatball. Place a cube of cheese in the center and form the ball around it.

Place the meatballs into the air fryer, working in batches if necessary. Adjust the temperature to 350 Degrees F and set the timer for 15 minutes

Meatballs will be slightly crispy on the outside and fully cooked when at least 180 Degrees F internally.

When they are finished cooking, toss the meatballs in the sauce and sprinkle with grated Parmesan for serving.

Nutrition: Calories: 447; Protein: 29.6g; Fiber: 1.8g; Fat: 29.7g; Carbs: 5.4g

261. Tuna Appetizer

Preparation Time: 15 minutes
Servings: 2

Ingredients:

1 lb. tuna, skinless; boneless and cubed

3 scallion stalks; minced

1 chili pepper; minced

2 tomatoes; cubed

1 tbsp. coconut aminos

2 tbsp. olive oil

1 tbsp. coconut cream

1 tsp. sesame seeds

Directions:

In a pan that fits your air fryer, mix all the ingredients except the sesame seeds, toss, introduce in the fryer and cook at 360°F for 10 minutes

Divide into bowls and serve as an appetizer with sesame seeds sprinkled on top.

Nutrition: Calories: 231; Fat: 18g; Fiber: 3g; Carbs: 4g; Protein: 18g

262. Cheese and Leeks Dip

Preparation Time: 17 minutes
Servings: 6

Ingredients:

2 spring onions; minced

4 leeks; sliced

¼ cup coconut cream

3 tbsp. coconut milk

2 tbsp. butter; melted

Salt and white pepper to the taste

Directions:

In a pan that fits your air fryer, mix all the ingredients and whisk them well.

Introduce the pan in the fryer and cook at 390°F for 12 minutes. Divide into bowls and serve

Nutrition: Calories: 204; Fat: 12g; Fiber: 2g; Carbs: 4g; Protein: 14g

263. Cucumber Salsa

Preparation Time: 10 minutes
Servings: 4

Ingredients:

1 ½ lb. cucumbers; sliced

2 red chili peppers; chopped.

2 tomatoes cubed

2 spring onions; chopped.

1 tbsp. balsamic vinegar

2 tbsp. ginger; grated

A drizzle of olive oil

Directions:

In a pan that fits your air fryer, mix all the ingredients, toss, introduce in the fryer and cook at 340°F for 5 minutes

Divide into bowls and serve cold as an appetizer.

Nutrition: Calories: 150; Fat: 2g; Fiber: 1g; Carbs: 2g; Protein: 4g

264. Chicken Cubes

Preparation Time: 25 minutes
Servings: 4

Ingredients:

1 lb. chicken breasts, skinless; boneless and cubed

2 eggs

¾ cup coconut flakes

2 tsp. garlic powder

Cooking spray

Salt and black pepper to taste.

Directions:

Put the coconut in a bowl and mix the eggs with garlic powder, salt and pepper in a second one.

Dredge the chicken cubes in eggs and then in coconut and arrange them all in your air fryer's basket

Grease with cooking spray, cook at 370°F for 20 minutes. Arrange the chicken bites on a platter and serve as an appetizer.

Nutrition: Calories: 202; Fat: 12g; Fiber: 2g; Carbs: 4g; Protein: 7g

265. Salmon Spread

Preparation Time: 11 minutes
Servings: 4

Ingredients:

8 oz. cream cheese, soft

½ cup coconut cream

4 oz. smoked salmon, skinless; boneless and minced

2 tbsp. lemon juice

1 tbsp. chives; chopped.

A pinch of salt and black pepper

Directions:

Take a bowl and mix all the ingredients and whisk them really well.

Transfer the mix to a ramekin, place it in your air fryer's basket and cook at 360°F for 6 minutes

Nutrition: Calories: 180; Fat: 7g; Fiber: 1g; Carbs: 5g; Protein: 7g

266. Crustless Pizza

Preparation Time: 10 minutes
Servings: 1

Ingredients:

2 slices sugar-free bacon; cooked and crumbled

7 slices pepperoni

½ cup shredded mozzarella cheese

¼ cup cooked ground sausage

2 tbsp. low-carb, sugar-free pizza sauce, for dipping

1 tbsp. grated Parmesan cheese

Directions:

Cover the bottom of a 6-inch cake pan with mozzarella. Place pepperoni, sausage and bacon on top of cheese and sprinkle with Parmesan

Place pan into the air fryer basket. Adjust the temperature to 400 Degrees F and set the timer for 5 minutes.

Remove when cheese is bubbling and golden. Serve warm with pizza sauce for dipping.

Nutrition: Calories: 466; Protein: 28.1g; Fiber: 0.5g; Fat: 34.0g; Carbs: 5.2g

267. Olives and Zucchini Cakes

Preparation Time: 17 minutes
Servings: 6

Ingredients:

3 spring onions; chopped.

½ cup kalamata olives, pitted and minced

3 zucchinis; grated

½ cup parsley; chopped.

½ cup almond flour

1 egg

Cooking spray

Salt and black pepper to taste.

Directions:

Take a bowl and mix all the ingredients except the cooking spray, stir well and shape medium cakes out of this mixture

Place the cakes in your air fryer's basket, grease them with cooking spray and cook at 380°F for 6 minutes on each side. Serve as an appetizer.

Nutrition: Calories: 165; Fat: 5g; Fiber: 2g; Carbs: 3g; Protein: 7g

268. Tomato Bites

Preparation Time: 25 minutes
Servings: 6

Ingredients:

6 tomatoes; halved

2 oz. watercress

3 oz. cheddar cheese; grated

1 tbsp. olive oil

3 tsp. sugar-free apricot jam

2 tsp. oregano; dried

A pinch of salt and black pepper

Directions:

Spread the jam on each tomato half, sprinkle oregano, salt and pepper and drizzle the oil all over them

Introduce them in the fryer's basket, sprinkle the cheese on top and cook at 360°F for 20 minutes

Arrange the tomatoes on a platter, top each half with some watercress and serve as an appetizer.

Nutrition: Calories: 131; Fat: 7g; Fiber: 2g; Carbs: 4g; Protein: 7g

269. Spinach Rolls

Preparation Time: 26 minutes
Servings: 6

Ingredients:

3 cups mozzarella; shredded

6 oz. spinach; chopped.

4 oz. cream cheese, soft

½ cup almond flour

2 eggs; whisked

¼ cup parmesan; grated

2 tbsp. ghee; melted

4 tbsp. coconut flour

A pinch of salt and black pepper

Directions:

Take a bowl and mix the mozzarella with coconut and almond flour, eggs, salt and pepper, stir well until you obtain a dough and roll it well on a parchment paper

Cut into triangles and leave them aside for now

Take a bowl and mix the spinach with parmesan, cream cheese, salt and pepper and stir really well.

Divide this into the center of each dough triangle, roll and seal the edges

Brush the rolls with the ghee, place them in your air fryer's basket and cook at 360°F for 20 minutes. Serve as an appetizer.

Nutrition: Calories: 210; Fat: 8g; Fiber: 1g; Carbs: 3g; Protein: 8g

270. Ranch Roasted Almonds

Preparation Time: 11 minutes
Servings: 2 cups

Ingredients:

½ (1-oz.ranch dressing mix packet

2 cups raw almonds.

2 tbsp. unsalted butter; melted.

Directions:

Take a large bowl, toss almonds in butter to evenly coat. Sprinkle ranch mix over almonds and toss. Place almonds into the air fryer basket

Adjust the temperature to 320 Degrees F and set the timer for 6 minutes. Shake the basket two or three times during cooking

Let cool at least 20 minutes. Almonds will be soft but become crunchier during cooling. Store in an airtight container up to 3 days.

Nutrition: Calories: 190; Protein: 6.0g; Fiber: 3.0g; Fat: 16.7g; Carbs: 7.0g

271. Pickled Snack

Preparation Time: 25 minutes
Servings: 4

Ingredients:

4 dill pickle spears; sliced in half and quartered

1 cup avocado mayonnaise

8 bacon slices; halved

Directions:

Wrap each pickle spear in a bacon slice, put them in your air fryer's basket and cook at 400°F for 20 minutes.

Serve as a snack with the mayonnaise

Nutrition: Calories: 100; Fat: 4g; Fiber: 2g; Carbs: 3g; Protein: 4g

272. Avocado Bites

Preparation Time: 13 minutes
Servings: 4

Ingredients:

4 avocados, peeled, pitted and cut into wedges

1 ½ cups almond meal

1 egg; whisked

A pinch of salt and black pepper

Cooking spray

Directions:

Put the egg in a bowl and the almond meal in another.

Season avocado wedges with salt and pepper, coat them in egg and then in meal almond

Arrange the avocado bites in your air fryer's basket, grease them with cooking spray and cook at 400°F for 8 minutes. Serve as a snack right away

Nutrition: Calories: 200; Fat: 12g; Fiber: 3g; Carbs: 5g; Protein: 16g

273. Asparagus Wraps

Preparation Time: 20 minutes
Servings: 8

Ingredients:

16 asparagus spears; trimmed

16 bacon strips

1 tbsp. lemon juice

2 tbsp. olive oil

1 tsp. oregano; chopped.

1 tsp. thyme; chopped.

A pinch of salt and black pepper

Directions:

Take a bowl and mix the oil with lemon juice, the herbs, salt and pepper and whisk well.

Brush the asparagus spears with this mix and wrap each in a bacon strip

Arrange the asparagus wraps in your air fryer's basket and cook at 390°F for 15 minutes.

Nutrition: Calories: 173; Fat: 4g; Fiber: 2g; Carbs: 3g; Protein: 6g

274. Warm Tomato Salsa

Preparation Time: 13 minutes
Servings: 4

Ingredients:

2 spring onions; chopped.

1 garlic clove; minced

4 tomatoes; cubed

3 chili peppers; minced

2 tbsp. lime juice

2 tsp. parsley; chopped.

2 tsp. cilantro; chopped.

Cooking spray

Directions:

Grease a pan that fits your air fryer with the cooking spray and mix all the ingredients inside.

Introduce the pan in the machine and cook at 360°F for 8 minutes. Divide into bowls and serve

Nutrition: Calories: 148; Fat: 1g; Fiber: 2g; Carbs: 3g; Protein: 5g

275. Zucchini Chips

Preparation Time: 20 minutes
Servings: 6

Ingredients:

3 zucchinis, thinly sliced

1 cup almond flour

2 eggs; whisked

Salt and black pepper to taste.

Directions:

Take a bowl and mix the eggs with salt and pepper. Put the flour in a second bowl.

Dredge the zucchinis in flour and then in eggs

Arrange the chips in your air fryer's basket, cook at 350°F for 15 minutes and serve as a snack.

Nutrition: Calories: 120; Fat: 4g; Fiber: 2g; Carbs: 3g; Protein: 5g

276. Parsley Meatballs

Preparation Time: 25 minutes
Servings: 6

Ingredients:

1 lb. beef meat, ground

2 tbsp. parsley; chopped.

1 tsp. onion powder

1 tsp. garlic powder

Cooking spray

A pinch of salt and black pepper

Directions:

Take a bowl and mix all the ingredients except the cooking spray, stir well and shape medium meatballs out of this mix

Pace them in your lined air fryer's basket, grease with cooking spray and cook at 360°F for 20 minutes

Nutrition: Calories: 180; Fat: 5g; Fiber: 2g; Carbs: 5g; Protein: 7g

277. Cheese Chips

Preparation Time: 7 minutes
Servings: 4

Ingredients:

8 oz. cheddar cheese; shredded

1 tsp. sweet paprika

Directions:

Divide the cheese in small heaps in a pan that fits the air fryer, sprinkle the paprika on top, introduce the pan in the machine and cook at 400°F for 5 minutes

Cool down the chips and serve them.

Nutrition: Calories: 150; Fat: 4g; Fiber: 3g; Carbs: 4g; Protein: 6g

278. Sweet Pepper Poppers

Preparation Time: 23 minutes
Servings: 16 halves

Ingredients:

8 mini sweet peppers

4 slices sugar-free bacon; cooked and crumbled

¼ cup shredded pepper jack cheese

4 oz. full-fat cream cheese; softened.

Directions:

Remove the tops from the peppers and slice each one in half lengthwise. Use a small knife to remove seeds and membranes

In a small bowl, mix cream cheese, bacon and pepper jack

Place 3 tsp. of the mixture into each sweet pepper and press down smooth. Place into the fryer basket. Adjust the temperature to 400 Degrees F and set the timer for 8 minutes. Serve warm.

Nutrition: Calories: 176; Protein: 7.4g; Fiber: 0.9g; Fat: 13.4g; Carbs: 3.6g

279. Bacon Wrapped Onion Rings.

Preparation Time: 15 minutes
Servings: 4

Ingredients:

1 large onion; peeled.

8 slices sugar-free bacon.

1 tbsp. sriracha

Directions:

Slice onion into ¼-inch-thick slices. Brush sriracha over the onion slices. Take two slices of onion and wrap bacon around the rings. Repeat with remaining onion and bacon

Place into the air fryer basket. Adjust the temperature to 350 Degrees F and set the timer for 10 minutes.

Use tongs to flip the onion rings halfway through the cooking time. When fully cooked, bacon will be crispy. Serve warm

Nutrition: Calories: 105; Protein: 7.5g; Fiber: 0.6g; Fat: 5.9g; Carbs: 4.3g

280. Zucchini Salsa

Preparation Time: 20 minutes
Servings: 6

Ingredients:

1 ½ lb. zucchinis, roughly cubed

2 tomatoes; cubed

2 spring onions; chopped.

1 tbsp. balsamic vinegar

Salt and black pepper to taste.

Directions:

In a pan that fits your air fryer, mix all the ingredients, toss, introduce the pan in the fryer and cook at 360°F for 15 minutes

Divide the salsa into cups and serve cold.

Nutrition: Calories: 164; Fat: 6g; Fiber: 2g; Carbs: 3g; Protein: 8g

281. Mushroom Platter

Preparation Time: 17 minutes
Servings: 4

Ingredients:

12 oz. Portobello mushrooms; sliced

2 tbsp. olive oil

2 tbsp. balsamic vinegar

½ tsp. rosemary; dried

½ tsp. thyme; dried

½ tsp. basil; dried

½ tsp. tarragon; dried

A pinch of salt and black pepper

Directions:

Take a bowl and mix all the ingredients and toss well.

Arrange the mushroom slices in your air fryer's basket and cook at 380°F for 12 minutes. Arrange the mushroom slices on a platter and serve

Nutrition: Calories: 147; Fat: 8g; Fiber: 2g; Carbs: 3g; Protein: 3g

282. Crab Balls

Preparation Time: 25 minutes
Servings: 8

Ingredients:

16 oz. lump crabmeat; chopped.

2/3 cup almond meal

½ cup coconut cream

1 egg; whisked

2 tbsp. chives, mined

1 tsp. lemon juice

1 tsp. mustard

A pinch of salt and black pepper

Cooking spray

Directions:

Take a bowl and mix all the ingredients except the cooking spray and stir well.

Shape medium balls out of this mix, place them in the fryer and cook at 390°F for 20 minutes

Nutrition: Calories: 141; Fat: 7g; Fiber: 2g; Carbs: 4g; Protein: 9g

283. Bacon Wrapped Brie

Preparation Time: 15 minutes
Servings: 8

Ingredients:

1 (8-oz.round Brie

4 slices sugar-free bacon.

Directions:

Place two slices of bacon to form an X. Place the third slice of bacon horizontally across the center of the X. Place the fourth slice of bacon vertically across the X. It should look like a plus sign (+on top of an X. Place the Brie in the center of the bacon

Wrap the bacon around the Brie, securing with a few toothpicks. Cut a piece of parchment to fit your air fryer basket and place the bacon-wrapped Brie on top. Place inside the air fryer basket.

Adjust the temperature to 400 Degrees F and set the timer for 10 minutes. When 3 minutes remain on the timer, carefully flip Brie

When cooked, bacon will be crispy and cheese will be soft and melty. To serve; cut into eight slices.

Nutrition: Calories: 116; Protein: 7.7g; Fiber: 0.0g; Fat: 8.9g; Carbs: 0.2g

284. Shrimp Balls

Preparation Time: 20 minutes
Servings: 4

Ingredients:

1 lb. shrimp, peeled, deveined and minced

1 egg; whisked

½ cup coconut flour

1 tbsp. avocado oil

3 tbsp. coconut; shredded

1 tbsp. cilantro; chopped.

Directions:

Take a bowl and mix all the ingredients, stir well and shape medium balls out of this mix.

Place the balls in your lined air fryer's basket, cook at 350°F for 15 minutes and serve

Nutrition: Calories: 184; Fat: 5g; Fiber: 2g; Carbs: 4g; Protein: 7g

Chapter 9. Desserts

285. Awesome Chinese Doughnuts

Preparation Time: 10 minutes

Cooking Time: 8 minutes

Servings: 8

Nutrition:

Calories: 259

Fat: 15.9 g

Carbs: 27 g

Protein: 3.8 g

Ingredients:

1 tbsp. baking powder

6 tbsps. coconut oil

¾ cup of coconut milk

2 tsps. sugar

2 cup all-purpose flour

½ tsp. sea salt

Directions:

Preheat the air fryer to 3500F.

Mix baking powder, flour, sugar, and salt in a bowl.

Add coconut oil and mix well. Add coconut milk and mix until well combined.

Knead dough for 3-4 minutes.

Roll dough half inch thick and using cookie cutter cut doughnuts.

Place doughnuts in cake pan and brush with oil. Place cake pan in air fryer basket and air fry doughnuts for 5 minutes. Turn doughnuts to other side and air fry for 3 minutes more.

Serve and enjoy.

286. Crispy Bananas

Preparation Time: 10 minutes

Cooking Time: 10 minutes

Servings: 4

Nutrition:

Calories: 282

Fat: 9 g

Carbs: 46 g

Protein: 5 g

Ingredients:

4 sliced ripe bananas

1 egg

½ cup breadcrumbs

1 ½ tbsps. cinnamon sugar

1 tbsp. almond meal

1 ½ tbsps. coconut oil

1 tbsp. crushed cashew

¼ cup corn flour

Directions:

Set the pan on fire to heat the coconut oil over medium heat and add breadcrumbs in the pan and stir for 3-4 minutes.

Remove pan from heat and transfer breadcrumbs in a bowl.

Add almond meal and crush cashew in breadcrumbs and mix well.

Dip banana half in corn flour then in egg and finally coat with breadcrumbs.

Place coated banana in air fryer basket. Sprinkle with Cinnamon Sugar.

Air fry at 350 F/ 176 C for 10 minutes.

Serve and enjoy.

287. Air-Fried Banana and Walnuts Muffins

Preparation Time: 10 minutes

Cooking Time: 10 minutes

Servings: 2

Nutrition:

Calories: 192

Fat: 12.3 g

Carbs: 19.4 g

Protein: 1.9 g

Ingredients:

¼ cup flour

½ tsp. baking powder

¼ cup mashed banana

¼ cup butter

1 tbsp. chopped walnuts

¼ cup oats

Directions:

Spray four muffin molds with cooking spray and set aside.

In a bowl, mix together mashed bananas, walnuts, sugar, and butter.

In another bowl, mix oat flour, and baking powder.

Combine the flour mixture to the banana mixture.

Pour batter into prepared muffin mold.

Place in air fryer basket and cook at 320 F/ 160 C for 10 minutes.

Remove muffins from air fryer and allow to cool completely.

Serve and enjoy.

288. Air-Fryer Blueberry Muffins

Preparation Time: 10 minutes

Cooking Time: 14 minutes

Servings: 2

Nutrition:

Calories: 435

Fat: 20.9 g

Carbs: 55 g

Protein: 9 g

Ingredients:

1/3 cup milk

2 tbsps. sugar

2/3 cup flour

¾ cup blueberries

3 tbsps. melted butter

1 egg

1 tsp. baking powder

Directions:

Spray four silicone muffin cups with cooking spray and set aside.

In a bowl, mix together all ingredients until well combined.

Pour batter into prepared muffin cups.

Place muffin cups in air fryer basket and cook at 320 F/ 160 C for 14 minutes.

Serve and enjoy.

289. Nutty Mix

Preparation Time: 5 minutes

Cooking Time: 4 minutes

Servings: 6

Nutrition:

Calories: 316

Fat: 29 g

Carbs: 11.3 g

Protein: 7.6 g

Ingredients:

2 cup mix nuts

1 tsp. ground cumin

1 tsp. chili powder

1 tbsp. melted butter

1 tsp. salt

1 tsp. pepper

Directions:

Set all ingredients in a large bowl and toss until well coated.

Preheat the air fryer at 3500F for 5 minutes.

Add mix nuts in air fryer basket and air fry for 4 minutes. Shake basket halfway through.

Serve and enjoy.

290. Vanilla Spiced Soufflé

Preparation Time: 20 minutes

Cooking Time: 32 minutes

Servings: 6

Nutrition:

Calories: 215

Fat: 12.2g

Carbs: 18.98g

Protein: 6.66g

Ingredients:

¼ cup all-purpose flour

1 cup whole milk

2 tsps. vanilla extract

1 tsp. cream of tartar

1 vanilla bean

4 egg yolks

1-oz. sugar

¼ cup softened butter

¼ cup sugar

5 egg whites

Directions:

Combine flour and butter in a bowl until the mixture becomes a smooth paste.

Set the pan over medium flame to heat the milk. Add sugar and stir until dissolved.

Mix in the vanilla bean and bring to a boil.

Beat the mixture using a wire whisk as you add the butter and flour mixture.

Lower the heat to simmer until thick. Discard the vanilla bean. Turn off the heat.

Place them on an ice bath and allow to cool for 10 minutes.

Grease 6 ramekins with butter. Sprinkle each with a bit of sugar.

Beat the egg yolks in a bowl. Add the vanilla extract and milk mixture. Mix until combined.

Whisk together the tartar cream, egg whites, and sugar until it forms medium stiff peaks.

Gradually fold egg whites into the soufflé base. Transfer the mixture to the ramekins.

Put 3 ramekins in the cooking basket at a time. Cook for 16 minutes at 330 degrees. Move to a wire rack for cooling and cook the rest.

Sprinkle powdered sugar on top and drizzle with chocolate sauce before serving.

291. Apricot Blackberry Crumble

Preparation Time: 10 minutes

Cooking Time: 20 minutes

Servings: 8

Nutrition:

Calories: 217

Fat: 7.44g

Carbs: 36.2g

Protein: 2.3g

Ingredients:

1 cup flour

18 oz. fresh apricots

5 tbsps. cold butter

½ cup sugar

5½ oz. fresh blackberries

Salt

2 tbsps. lemon juice

Directions:

Put the apricots and blackberries in a bowl. Add lemon juice and 2 tbsps. of sugar. Mix until combined.

Transfer the mixture to a baking dish.

Put flour, the rest of the sugar, and a pinch of salt in a bowl. Mix well. Add a tbsp. of cold butter.

Combine the mixture until it becomes crumbly. Put this on top of the fruit mixture and press it down lightly.

Set the baking tray in the cooking basket.

Cook for 20 minutes at 390 degrees.

Allow to cool before slicing and serving.

292. Chocolate Cup cakes

Preparation Time: 5 minutes

Cooking Time: 12 minutes

Servings: 6

Nutrition:

Calories: 289

Protein: 8.72 g

Fat: 11.5 g

Carbs: 38.94 g

Ingredients:

3 eggs

¼ cup caster sugar

¼ cup cocoa powder

1 tsp. baking powder

1 cup milk

¼ tsp. vanilla essence

2 cup all-purpose flour

4 tbsps. butter

Directions:

Preheat your Air Fryer to a temperature of 400°F (200°C).

Beat eggs with sugar in a bowl until creamy.

Add butter and beat again for 1-2 minutes.

Now add flour, cocoa powder, milk, baking powder, and vanilla essence, mix with a spatula.

Fill ¾ of muffin tins with the mixture and place them into Air Fryer basket.

Let cook for 12 minutes.

Serve!

293. Stuffed Baked Apples

Preparation Time: 3 minutes

Cooking Time: 12 minutes

Servings: 4

Nutrition:

Calories: 324

Protein: 2.8 g

Fat: 6.99 g

Carbs: 70.31 g

Ingredients:

4 tbsps. honey

¼ cup brown sugar

½ cup raisins

½ cup crushed walnuts

4 large apples

Directions:

Preheat Air Fryer to a temperature of 350°F (180°C).

Cut the apples from the stem and remove the inner using spoon.

Now fill each apple with raisins, walnuts, honey, and brown sugar.

Transfer apples in a pan and place in Air Fryer basket, cook for 12 minutes.

Serve.

294. Roasted Pineapples with Vanilla Zest

Preparation Time: 5 minutes

Cooking Time: 8 minutes

Servings: 4

Nutrition:

Calories: 90

Protein: 0.79 g

Fat: 0.17 g

Carbs: 23.22 g

Ingredients:

2 anise stars

¼ cup orange juice

1 tsp. lime juice

1 vanilla pod

2 tbsps. caster sugar

¼ cup pineapple juice

1 lb. pineapple slices

Directions:

Preheat Air Fryer to a temperature of 350°F (180°C).

Take a baking pan that can fit into Air Fryer basket.

Now add pineapple juice, sugar, orange juice, anise stars, and vanilla pod into a pan and mix well.

Place in pineapple slices evenly and transfer pan into Air Fryer basket.

Cook for 8 minutes.

Serve!

295. Vanilla Coconut Pie

Preparation Time: 15 minutes

Cooking Time: 12 minutes

Servings: 4

Nutrition:

Calories: 272

Fat: 27 g

Carbs: 7.8 g

Protein: 5.3 g

Ingredients:

Shredded coconut, 1 cup

Granulated monk fruit, ½ cup

Vanilla extract, 1 ½ tsps.

Eggs, 2.

Almond milk, 1 ½ cup

Coconut flour, ½ cup

Butter, ¼ cup

Directions:

Combine all the ingredients in a suitable mixing bowl using a wooden spatula to form a batter.

Pour this batter into a 6-inch pie pan then place this pan in the air fryer basket.

Return the basket to the air fryer then cook the pie for 12 minutes at 3700 F on Air Fry Mode.

Allow it to cool then serve.

296. Cookie Dough Ball

Preparation Time: 15 minutes

Cooking Time: 5 minutes

Servings: 4

Nutrition:

Calories: 179

Fat: 10.7 g

Carbs: 24.2 g

Protein: 6.9 g

Ingredients:

Vanilla extract, ½ tsp.

Swerve sugar substitute, 1 tbsp.

Egg, 1.

Mini sugar-free chocolate chips, 3 tbsps.

Coconut flour, ½ cup

Xanthan gum, ¼ tsp.

Coconut oil.

Baking powder, ½ tsp.

Almond flour, ½ cup

Trivia sugar substitute, ½ tbsp.

Melted butter, ½ tbsp.

Cinnamon, ¼ tsp.

Directions:

In a mixing bowl, incorporate all the ingredients.

Whisk in egg, vanilla, and melted butter.

Mix well until a smooth dough forms then fold in chocolate chips.

Roll the dough into a ball then refrigerate until air fryer is ready.

Grease the air fryer basket with coconut oil and preheat the fryer to 375 degrees F.

Divide the dough into cookie-sized balls and place them in the basket.

Set the basket back to the air fryer and cook them for 5 minutes on Air Fry Mode.

Serve.

297. Pumpkin Bread Cake

Preparation Time: 15 minutes

Cooking Time: 25 minutes

Servings: 6

Nutrition:

Calories: 84

Fat: 3.7 g

Carbs: 9.1 g

Protein: 3.6 g

Ingredients:

Pumpkin puree, ¼ cup

Large brown eggs, 2.

Pumpkin pie spice mix, 1 tsp.

Stevia, 2 tsps.

Vanilla extract, 1 tsp.

Himalayan pink salt, 1/8 tsp.

Unsweetened almond milk, 2 tbsps.

Organic coconut flour, ¼ cup

Baking powder, 1 tsp.

Directions:

Whisk eggs with almond milk, pumpkin puree, and vanilla in a mixer.

Mix in the remaining ingredients to incorporate until smooth.

Spread this batter into a 7-inch pan lined with parchment paper.

Move the pan to the air fryer basket and return the basket to the fryer.

Cook the cake batter for 25 minutes at 3500 F on Air Fry Mode.

Slice after cooling to serve

298. Air Fried Beignets

Preparation Time: 15 minutes

Cooking Time: 5 minutes

Servings: 4

Nutrition:

Calories: 114

Fat: 9 g

Carbs: 7.1 g

Protein: 3.7 g

Ingredients:

Almond flour, 1 ½ cup

Coconut milk, ½ cup

Egg, 1.

Vanilla extract, 1 tbsp.

Salt, ¼ tsp.

Swerve sugar substitute, 3 tbsps.

Cornstarch, ¼ tsp.

Swerve confectioner sugar substitute

Butter, 1 tbsp.

Cooking oil

Directions:

Mix almond flour with salt, and cornstarch in a suitable bowl.

Heat milk in the microwave then mix it with Swerve and butter.

Once slightly cooled, whisk in vanilla and egg.

Combine the flour mixture and milk mixture with a hand blender.

Cover this batter and refrigerate it for 30 minutes.

Grease the air fryer basket with cooking oil and drop the batter into the basket using an ice cream scoop.

Add more scoops with sufficient distance in between, spray these balls with cooking oil.

Set the basket back to the air fryer and cook the beignets for 5 minutes at 3300 F on Air Fry Mode.

Serve once cooled and garnish with Swerve confectioner's sugar substitute.

299. Chocolate Mayo Cake

Preparation Time: 15 minutes

Cooking Time: 2 minutes

Servings: 2

Nutrition:

Calories: 239

Fat: 17.1 g

Carbs: 4.2 g

Protein: 6.9 g

Ingredients:

Large egg, 1.

Water, 2 tbsps.

Swerve sugar substitute, 3 tbsps.

Dark cocoa powder, 2 tbsps.

Mayonnaise, ¼ cup

Vanilla extract, ½ tsp.

Cooking oil

Baking powder, 1 tsp.

Almond flour, 4 tbsps.

Coconut flour, 1½ tbsps.

Directions:

Combine the dry ingredients in a 4-cup mixing bowl.

Whisk in the remaining ingredients to create a smooth batter.

Divide the batter into two 4-ounce ramekins, greased with cooking oil.

Place the ramekins in the air fryer basket and return the basket to the air fryer.

Cook them for 2 minutes on air fry mode at 3500 F.

Garnish with whipped cream.

Serve.

Chapter 10. 21-day meal plan

DAY	BREAKFAST	MAINS	SNACK/DESSERT
1.	Peppery Sausage & Parsley Patties	Chicken Coconut Meatballs	Spinach Rolls
2.	Air Fried Mac and Cheese	Smoked Lamb Chops	Ranch Roasted Almonds
3.	Prosciutto & Mozzarella Crostini	Herbed Lamb	Avocado Bites
4.	Vanilla Lemon Cheesecake	BBQ Chicken Wings	Cheese Chips
5.	Cinnamon Baked Apples with Raisins & Walnuts	Spicy Mexican Chicken Burgers	Zucchini Chips
6.	Vanilla Chocolate Brownies with Walnuts	Beef Lasagna	Warm Tomato Salsa
7.	Raspberry Chocolate Cake	Beef Satay	Asparagus Wraps
8.	Amazing Marshmallows Pie	Coffee & Spice Ribeye Steak	Pickled Snack
9.	Caramel Apple & Cinnamon Cake	Lentils Stew	Parsley Meatballs
10.	Blueberry & Yogurt Cups	Cheesy Chicken and Zucchini	Sweet Pepper Poppers
11.	Honeyed White Chocolate Cake	Shrimp Stew	Bacon Wrapped Onion Rings

12.	Coconut Oat Cookies Filled with White Chocolate	Beef Meatballs Bowls	Shrimp Balls
13.	Orange & Chocolate Fudge with Honey Icing	Salmon Meatballs	Cookie Dough Ball
14.	Vanilla Crème Caramel	Balsamic Cod Mix	Pumpkin Bread Cake
15.	Tasty Choco-Banana Sandwich	Sausage Pan	Roasted Pineapples with Vanilla Zest
16.	Homemade Orange Curd	Lemony Chicken Wings	Chocolate Cup cakes
17.	Dreamy White Chocolate Dessert	Buffalo Chicken Legs	Stuffed Baked Apples
18.	Dark Chocolate & Peanut Butter Fondant	Jalapeno Popper Stuffed Chicken Breast	Vanilla Coconut Pie
19.	Delicious Figs with Honey & Mascarpone	BBQ Pork Bowls	Air Fried Beignets
20.	Marshmallows Choco S´mores	Turkey Breast	Chocolate Mayo Cake
21.	Creamy Yogurt & Lime Muffins	Pork and Potatoes Mix	Apricot Blackberry Crumble

Conclusion

I hope this book was able to help you to understand the benefits of an Air Fryer and the basics on how to use it. The next step is to plan your meals and gather the ingredients. This appliance is easy to use and you will eventually get the hang of the process. Once you have tried several recipes, you can already start tweaking the ingredients to create variations or start making your own.

Enjoy the process of preparing your meals in a healthier way using this innovation when it comes to cooking.